More Praise for *101 Optimal Life Foods*

"The world needs more dietitians like David—he loves food *and* nutrition. Your copy of *101 Optimal Life Foods* can be your best medicine."

—JOHN LA PUMA, MD, director, Santa Barbara Institute for Medical Nutrition and Healthy Weight, and co-author of *ChefMD's Big Book of Culinary Medicine* and *The RealAge Diet*

"This book explains how to incorporate functional foods into our daily diets; it's a must-read for everyone who wants to eat well and feel great!"

—JAMES PAINTER, PhD, RD, chair, School of Family and Consumer Sciences, Eastern Illinois University

Praise for *101 Foods That Could Save Your Life*

"We are in a new era in nutrition, one that has dietitians telling us what to eat for better health instead of what not to eat. That is why... *101 Foods That Could Save Your Life*... is important."

—*The Dallas Morning News*

"This fascinating look at food as therapy is an A–Z guide to common nuts, seeds, fruits, vegetables, herbs, and grains with uncommon powers."

—*BookPage*

"This book not only tells you what to eat but why.... Everything is written in short, easily digestible blurbs so you don't have to finish the whole thing in one sitting. But you just might want to once you get started."

—*Fort Worth Star-Telegram*

"For the millions of Americans tired of hearing about 'what not to eat,' this book is a refreshing and enlightening guide to improving your health by *adding* delicious foods to your diet. Dave's simple explanations for why these foods are potential 'life savers' makes the book enjoyable to read, and the recipes bring the science to life on your plate."

—CYNTHIA SASS, MPH, RD, nutrition director, *Prevention* magazine

"Dave Grotto goes far beyond telling you what's good for you, why it's good for you, and how much is good for you; he does so in a compelling, fun, nonpreachy, 'your best friend told you so' sort of way. *101 Foods* is a great book to have on the shelf."

—BRIAN WANSINK, PhD, director, Cornell University Food and Brand Lab, and author of *Mindless Eating*

ALSO BY DAVID GROTTO, RD, LDN

101 Foods That Could Save Your Life

101
OPTIMAL
LIFE FOODS

101
OPTIMAL
LIFE FOODS

DAVID GROTTO, RD, LDN

FOREWORD BY MONTEL WILLIAMS

BANTAM BOOKS

New York

The information found in this book is intended to help guide you toward healthier eating choices, but is not intended to replace the services of a qualified medical professional. Seek medical attention if you suspect that you have a health challenge.

Any mention of a particular organization, product, service, company, or professional does not imply endorsement by either the author or the publisher. Any adverse effect arising from the use or misuse of the information from this book is the sole responsibility of the reader and not that of the author or publisher.

Published in the United States by Bantam Books, an imprint of The Random House Publishing Group, a division of Random House, Inc., New York.

BANTAM BOOKS and the rooster colophon are registered trademarks of Random House, Inc.

Library of Congress Cataloging-in-Publication Data
Grotto, David W.
101 optimal life foods / by David Grotto ; foreword by Montel Williams.
        p. cm.
Includes bibliographical references and index.
ISBN 978-0-553-38626-4
1. Nutrition. 2. Natural foods. 3. Diet therapy. I. Title. II. Title: One hundred one optimal life foods. III. Title: One hundred and one optimal life foods.
RA784.G766 2010
613—dc22
2009035954

Printed in the United States of America

www.bantamdell.com

2 4 6 8 9 7 5 3 1

Book design by Diane Hobbing

To
my daughters,
Chloe,
Katie,
and
Madison,
whom
I simply adore

ACKNOWLEDGMENTS

I wish to express my sincere appreciation to the many kind friends, colleagues, and organizations that were instrumental in the creation of this book—whether through perspiration or inspiration!

To my wonderful research assistants, Jamie Bommarito, MS, RD; Karin Testa, MS, RD; Carolyn Tampe, MS, RD; and Brad Hirt, MS, RD: thank you for the countless hours of valuable research for this project. To my expert advisers—Gary Jay Barsky, MD; Christine Gerbstadt, MD, RD; Cynthia Sass, MPH, MA, RD, CSSD; Bonnie Taub-Dix, MA, RD; Carmina McGee, MS, RD; Leslie Bonci, MPH, RD; Elizabeth Somer, MA, RD; Tara Gidus, MS, RD; and Angela Grassi, MS, RD—your cutting-edge input was a huge asset to this book. Thank you!

And what is good nutrition without great taste? Not long lasting, that's for sure! Thank you, Chef J. Hugh McEvoy, for all of your support since the beginning, and to my other recipe contributors: Mindy Hermann, MBA, RD; Almond Board of California and the folks at Porter Novelli; Bell Brands; Connie Guttersen, PhD, RD; Bush Brothers; Chilean Avocado Importers Association; California Dried Plum Board and the folks at Ketchum; Chef Owen Tilley; Chef Sean O'Brien; Chef Elizabeth Wiley; Chef Cheryl Bell, MS,

RD; Chef Gail Roloff; Chef Robin Kirby; Justin Kubica; Mary Corlett and her staff at CHOW; Christine Gerbstadt, MD, RD; Cherry Marketing Institute; Deb Schiff; Diana Dyer, MS, RD; Chef Don Zajac; Chef Carrie Walters and all the folks at Dorothy Lane Market; Chef Elisa Hunziker; Sue McCloskey; Chef Scott Peacock; Georgia Pecan Commission; Sahlman Williams; Chef Jennifer Carden; all the folks at Lockheed Martin; Chef Spike Mendelsohn; Jennette Fulda; Quaker Oats and the folks at Olgivy; Roni Noone at Green Lite Bites; SOYJOY; California Strawberry Commission; Chef Jon Ashton (aka "Cheeky Monkey"); Chef Brian Stapleton; Vidalia Onion Committee; Washington Red Raspberry Commission; Welch's and the folks at Tonic; and last but not least, my wife, Sharon, for making it all come alive on the plate!

Very special thanks to those behind the scenes who have been so supportive of me, my family, and this project: Cathy Kapica, PhD, RD; Dee Munson; Katleen Bertoloni; Molly Spence; Steven McCauly; Mary Christ Irwin; Kathleen Zelman, MS, RD, and her colleagues at WebMD; Mike Farrah; Gary Calaroso; Mike and Sue McCloskey; my literary agent, Rick Broadhead; my editor, Philip Rappaport; all my colleagues at the American Dietetic Association; and my dear friend and agent, Beth Shepard, for her tireless support behind me and my work.

I also pay homage to my dearest lifelong friend, Paul Eckenstein, who has always told me what I needed (but not necessarily wanted) to hear. And thanks to all of my other friends and family, who are always so supportive.

Lastly, to my lovely daughters, Chloe, Katie, and Madison, and my beautiful wife, Sharon, whom I absolutely cherish and adore—thank you from the bottom of my heart, for without you, none of this would have been possible.

FOREWORD

You are holding a powerful book in your hands.

David Grotto is one of the best authorities on health and nutrition in the United States today, and he has written a groundbreaking guide for you to live your ultimate, optimal life—by eating delicious foods.

In seventeen years as a TV talk show host, I've had literally thousands of experts on my show, many of them doctors, scientists, and other health professionals. Of them, few have impressed me more than David Grotto. I respect and admire Dave a great deal, because he has a passion and an enthusiasm for seeking out the best research, science, and information to help you and me live better lives.

I think Dave Grotto's principles of enjoying delicious food as a pathway to magnificent health are fantastic, and I live by them every day.

Isn't it amazing how many health challenges can surprise us in the course of everyday life?

Out of nowhere, we can be hit with such maladies as fatigue, stress, pain, depression, cramps, headaches, arthritis, muscle aches, low libido, heartburn, and insomnia. They can sap our energy, waste our time, interfere with our quality of life, and prevent us from living the lives we deserve to live.

With *101 Optimal Life Foods,* Dave Grotto shows us how to use food to combat these ailments and fully enjoy our lives so we can grow and flourish.

In my case, I have a chronic disease called multiple sclerosis, and that means I live with pain, and with limitations. But I've learned that by following the Dave Grotto philosophy—basing my diet on lots of vegetables and fruits, healthy carbohydrates, and healthy fats—I can energize my body and soul, boost my mood, and perform at a much higher level of intensity in all areas of my life. This style of living well is exactly what the best experts recommend to everyone interested in fighting a number of chronic diseases, and to everyone interested in improving their overall health and longevity.

In this book, Dave drills down to the common, frustrating health challenges that can interfere with our living well every day, takes the latest scientific research breakthroughs on specific foods and supplements, and makes these insights come alive on our plates.

There is a bewildering array of information on health and nutrition out there, and a staggering number of people putting themselves forward as experts on health, diet, and nutrition. The world is filled with self-described health gurus, and doctors and nutritionists with shaky credentials who happen to have a diet book on the market hyping a secret ingredient or a restrictive diet program.

Dave Grotto is head and shoulders above the pack. He is a member of a select breed of nutritionists, those with the RD credential. It stands for "registered dietitian." That means that he has had rigorous training and a thorough grounding in the hard-core science of nutrition. He is committed to the rigors of research, to putting nutrition ideas to the scientific test. He has over twenty years of clinical experience helping people like you and me live healthier, more enjoyable, more productive lives.

What's also really impressive about Dave is that he was selected by the American Dietetic Association (ADA) to serve as their national media spokesman. This was a prestigious appointment, since the ADA is the world's largest organization of food and nutrition professionals, with more than 70,000 members committed to improving the nation's health.

In preparing this book, Dave has drawn not only on decades of clinical experience, but also on his consultations with some of the world's leading experts in medicine and nutrition.

It is great to have a guy like Dave Grotto on your team, to help you navigate your way through good and bad information, and to chart your course toward a rich, healthy life.

Almost 2,500 years ago, Hippocrates, the father of medicine, declared, "Let your food be your medicine and your medicine be your food." But in our current medical mind-set, the temptation for both doctors and patients is to immediately leap to drugs to fix our health problems. Doctors tend to reach for the prescription pad first as a knee-jerk reaction to the presentation of disease. Some of that certainly has to do with vastly more money being poured into pharmaceutical research than into food research.

I also think there's a basic sentiment in the medical community that underestimates the ability of people to make change in their lives. Doctors see the growing obesity epidemic and they think, "Why even bother to tell people to change their diet or lifestyle? Let's sign them right up for gastric bypass surgery or put them on medication." But if we really dig deep and drill down, there is good, credible research that shows that if we can make the effort to do it, improving our diets and lifestyles can have a huge impact on our lives.

Of course, we need drugs and we need doctors. But the other half of the equation is what we put into our bodies—the food patterns that can make us feel bad or make us feel magnificent.

Dave Grotto's philosophy is very much in line with mine. He promotes sustainable, commonsense, and research-based ways of tackling some of the tough day-to-day health challenges that you and I face. He and I don't believe in restrictive diets and fad diets. For most people, they simply don't work over the long haul. Dave believes not in focusing on what foods to avoid, but in celebrating the tremendous power of *adding* foods that help us be healthy, happy, and strong.

Dave believes in the pure pleasure of food, and the amazing power it has to address many of our health problems and to boost our positive mood and happiness.

With the mouthwatering recipes and convenient three-day menu plans in this book, Dave proves that healthy eating can and should be about pleasure.

101 Optimal Life Foods has the power to help you supercharge your health, feel great, and achieve your maximum potential every day. It is a book that is authoritative, illuminating, and filled with terrific ideas for you and your family to enjoy.

What does an optimal life mean to you?

To me, an optimal life is one where I have the freedom to live well, to achieve anything that is possible for my mind and body to achieve. It means that no physical or mental obstacle will prevent me from living a beautiful life with my friends and family.

It means flourishing mentally, emotionally, and physically.

You and I deserve an optimal life—a life filled with health, love, physical joy, and delicious food. And thanks to Dave Grotto, we now have a delicious new way to get there.

Montel Williams

CONTENTS

INTRODUCTION

Are You Living Optimally?

The latest trend surveys indicate that Americans are complaining more about their health than ever before. According to these surveys, baby boomers are ranking life's inconveniences and general feelings of malaise above serious life-or-death health issues.

For most of my career as a registered dietitian, I have seen hundreds if not thousands of patients who needed help fighting diseases that are considered life threatening. But over the past decade or so, I have been seeing more and more patients who are asking me for advice on how to improve the quality of their lives, first. Sure, they're still concerned about not dying from cancer, heart disease, diabetes, and the like, but they seem even more concerned about the troublesome manifestations of those diseases and side effects of their treatment regimens that can result in pain, fatigue, diarrhea, constipation, and so forth. For others, it is suffering from those pesky challenges that get in the way of "living," like arthritis, irritable bowel syndrome, and migraine headaches. But most interesting to me is that I'm seeing a greater percentage of patients who are faced with the unpleasant realities that come with getting older: physical-, mental-, and sexual-performance decline.

Optimal physical performance can be as simple as enjoying the company of family and friends without pain or having enough energy to get out and throw the ball around with your kids. Maybe it's falling asleep when you're supposed to or simply enjoying the food you eat without having to pay the consequences with acid blockers, laxatives, or antidiarrheals. Optimal mental performance can be as simple as not forgetting the names of people you see often or remembering where you left your keys last. What is wanted of sexual performance probably doesn't need further explanation here, but many of my patients would feel they were living optimally if they could be intimate with their spouses without the aid of pharmaceuticals or other assistance.

Though the precise definition of an *optimal life* may vary from one person to another, one thing we can agree on is that a life absent disease while also abundant with satisfactory performance is highly desirable. We've made great strides in extending life span during the last century, but in meaningful ways, boomers are not living quite as well as their parents. Alzheimer's, senile dementia, poor cognition, chronic heartburn, profound fatigue, stress, and poor physical, mental, and sexual performance are common twenty-first-century complaints.

Viagra, Cialis, and other modern miracle drugs that were developed to correct sexual dysfunction in the elderly are not only being prescribed and sold in record numbers to aging boomers, but also being prescribed to Gen Xers. Physiologically, forty-something and thirty-something men aren't supposed to need medicinal help achieving erections.

A few years ago, I put Chicago-area firefighters on a cholesterol-reduction program. As I recounted in *101 Foods That Could Save Your Life,* the participants, young and old alike, confided in me that they were feeling stressed, battling fatigue, and packing on pounds, even though they were reportedly eating the same amount of food they consumed in their youth. But once the firefighters started following my advice for lowering their cholesterol levels, they said they experienced better physical, mental, and sexual energy. And several confided that they were *really* happy about the latter!

I researched this phenomenon and found that many of the recommended foods that targeted cholesterol buildup in the arteries that feed the heart were at the same time widening blood passageways that feed the brain, muscles, and sex organs. For these firefighters, the *101 Foods* program was not only saving their lives, but helping them achieve optimal lives, too.

Many of today's health-related books claim that weight gain is the primary cause of our skyrocketing levels of stress and fatigue. But what came first? Are we tired because we're fat or are we fat because we're tired? There is good research that supports the latter hypothesis, but in reality, it is a combination of both. Unfortunately, our present medical model wants to recognize only the "tired because we're fat" part of the obesity equation. According to an excellent study from the University of Pennsylvania, stress and fatigue increase the drive to overconsume calorically dense foods that can lead to weight gain.

Are you shortchanging yourself a few hours of sleep most nights? If so, you're making it even harder to fully enjoy the waking hours. Researchers found that women who slept five or fewer hours per night were 32 percent more likely to gain weight and 15 percent more prone to becoming obese than those who got seven or more hours of shut-eye. Unfortunately for many, even if they try to go to bed earlier or sleep later, insomnia and other sleep disorders still afflict more than half of American adults. (And adolescent sleep deprivation complaints are on the rise, too.)

There is a way out of this morass that does not include obsessively counting calories or taking sleeping pills. In the pages that follow, you'll learn about foods that promote good sleeping habits. For example, the amino acid tryptophan, combined with carbohydrates, helps to jump-start production of the brain chemical serotonin, which promotes sleep (although it is better known for its effect on depression). You don't need to take tryptophan in a pill; it is present in dairy, lean meats such as chicken and turkey, eggs, soy, and peanut butter. When foods rich in this amino acid are combined with foods such as cereal, pasta, and potatoes, the sleep-promoting potential is something to dream about. Another "natural" sleep aid is melatonin, a naturally occurring hormone that helps regulate our biological clocks and is found in foods such as tart cherries and walnuts.

Good sleep is just one of the benefits that come with eating the great foods I discuss in this book. Beyond the sheer pleasure of enjoying what you eat, there are many foods that can improve your mood. By stimulating brain chemicals called neurotransmitters, many foods can reduce the effects of depression and anxiety, bringing joy to both your taste buds and your soul.

The examples above are just the tip of the iceberg. You'll discover why

- Fish rich in omega-3 fats, like salmon, seasoned with the Indian spice turmeric, can block inflammation pathways and reduce pain.
- Oatmeal and blueberries in the morning can improve cognitive function.
- Onions, rich in the plant chemical quercetin, along with mushrooms, which are among the richest food sources of vitamin D, improve the skeletal system of your body by driving calcium into your bones.
- Artichoke leaves contain powerful substances that help relax a spastic bowel naturally.
- Fermented foods such as yogurt, kefir, sauerkraut, miso, and kimchi are rich in friendly probiotic bacteria that keep irritable bowel syndrome flare-ups at bay.

How to Use This Book

101 Optimal Life Foods has the same "easy and fun read" format of *101 Foods That Could Save Your Life*. But this time, instead of an A–Y list of foods, the book is organized by "health challenge" categories. Each listing will contain helpful information about the health issue and what you can do about it naturally.

I've split *101 Optimal Life Foods* into two sections. The first covers seven distinct health challenges, including aging and damaged skin, circulatory problems, and declining mental, physical, and sexual/reproductive functioning. The second section gathers together dozens of delicious, nutritious recipes that make use (and often combine two or more) of the powerhouse foods in the book. Each entry in the first section discusses, in basic terms, what each condition is and what some of the common causes behind it are. I list foods that may actually worsen the condition and, of course, highlight foods that may help make it better.

As a registered dietitian, I have always been and continue to be about "food first." That will never change. However, dietary supplements alongside a healthy diet can also contribute to overall wellness. You'll find a list of supplements to try (and of those to avoid) for each health challenge.

You will also find three-day menu plans to get you started incorporating the 101 foods. Each menu plan includes three meals and two snacks and averages about 2,000 calories per day (with calorie counts listed in parentheses). I want you to try eating every three to four hours, which research shows is the best eating style for controlling your appetite and supplying you with enough consistent energy to meet your needs. You may need to add an additional snack between breakfast and lunch, especially if you are hungry or there is more than four hours between the two meals. Feel free to omit the evening snack if you are not hungry or eat a late dinner. Of course, the portion sizes can also be reduced or increased to meet your individual calorie needs. Keep in mind that the menu plan is just a suggestion to get you started, and that you can most certainly tweak it as you see fit.

The recommendations herein draw on my more than two decades of clinical experience as well as my interviews with some of the world's leading experts in medicine and nutrition. Besides my tips and raves, you will also be reading some of theirs.

I received such great feedback on the recipes from *101 Foods That Could Save Your Life* that it was apparent many of you were amazed at how great good health tastes. My "Taste rules!" approach incorporates recipes from a variety of culinary experts. The contributors include not only world-class chefs but also moms and dads who face the daily challenge of running their own "restaurants" and feeding their young ones nutritiously and deliciously. Of course, my lovely wife, Sharon, has whipped up a few of her own creations for you, too.

Get ready to take charge of your life and begin "living" again. I think you will find quite a few tools in *101 Optimal Life Foods* to help you rise to meet those challenges to *living optimally*.

SECTION ONE

THIRTY CHALLENGES
TO AN OPTIMAL LIFE

PART 1

THE SKIN YOU'RE IN

AGING AND DAMAGED SKIN

That Youthful Appearance

Did you know...*the effects of aging on the skin can be visibly apparent as early as the twenties?*

Optimal Food/Nutrient Highlights

Vitamin A−, E−, and C− rich foods, chocolate, apples, beans, tea, olive oil, vegetables, dried plums.

What Is Aging and Damaged Skin?

The skin is the body's first line of defense against environmental damage and foreign invaders such as harmful bacteria. Yet for all the protection the skin's three layers provide, if the skin isn't well cared for, the wear and tear of a well-lived life can leave one looking ravaged—not ravishing. Collagen and elastin form in the skin's middle layer, called the dermis. These two proteins give the skin firmness and the ability to stretch and bounce back into shape. The signs of aging become noticeable as collagen and elastin diminish and change over time.

Though skin cells constantly regenerate, the combination of genetics, environmental stressors, lifestyle, and the quality of our nutrition ultimately affects the rate at which our skin ages. The aging process begins around our mid-twenties, as collagen production slows and the elastin begins to lose its "spring." The rate of skin aging varies from individual to individual. As you and your skin age, you may begin to notice fine wrinkles; thin and transparent skin; loss of fat underneath the skin, which gives a "hollowed cheek and eye socket" appearance; sagging skin; or dry, itchy skin.

What Causes Premature Aging of the Skin?

Enemy #1: Sun exposure. Most premature aging of the skin is attributed to extrinsic or external factors over which we may have some influence. Repeated ultraviolet (UV) exposure breaks down collagen, impairs the synthesis of new collagen, and breaks down elastin. Not only do these processes cause the skin to become loose, wrinkled, and leathery, but UV exposure is associated with skin conditions like age spots, spider veins, and skin cancer.

Sun exposure is the biggest concern, yet there are other, unavoidable natural factors that can speed up wrinkling of the skin:

Repetitive facial expressions. What was once thought to help sagging facial muscles may actually lead to fine lines and wrinkles. As the skin ages, it loses its elasticity, and the "smile lines" that once disappeared when the smile went away can now show up as fine lines and wrinkles on the face. This is no excuse not to smile, because experts agree that nothing looks worse than a sad, *boo-hoo* face!

Sleeping position. Wrinkles can develop from sleeping on your side with your face on the pillow. Change your sleeping position if you can.

Gravity literally drags skin down over a lifetime.

Lifestyle. The choices that we make in our daily lives contribute to prematurely aging skin. The top three culprits are smoking, poor sleep habits, and poor or improper diet.

- *Smoking.* Like overexposure to the sun, smoking can cause the skin to age rapidly. Several studies compared people who smoke ten or more cigarettes daily for at least ten years with non-smokers. The results showed that the ten-a-day smokers' skin tended to be more deeply wrinkled and leathery.
- *Poor sleep habits.* Insufficient or poor-quality sleep is most noticeable on the face with dark circles and baggy eyes. In most cases, this appearance can be lessened by improving your sleep habits.
- *Poor or improper diet.* The skin requires adequate nutrition and hydration to keep it healthy in appearance and function.

Optimal Life Foods

Vitamins A, E, and C help the skin heal and repair itself and also help protect it from the ravages of ultraviolet light. Vitamin C is also essential for collagen production, which keeps skin firm.

Vitamin A–rich foods include eggs, milk, carrots, apricots, nectarines, sweet potatoes, and spinach.

Vitamin E–rich foods include almonds, sunflower seeds, avocados, olives, wheat germ, canola oil, and peanuts.

Vitamin C–rich foods include many common fruits like oranges, grapefruit, lemons, limes, kiwis, and cantaloupe; other semitropical and tropical fruits such as pomegranates, papaya, mangoes, guavas, and passion fruit; berries (strawberries, blackberries, elderberries); and vegetables like green and red peppers, broccoli, Brussels sprouts, tomatoes, potatoes, romaine lettuce, onions, cauliflower, kale, artichokes, fennel, cabbage, and chard. Researchers in the United Kingdom looked at vitamin C intake in 4,025 women and found that those who ate more vitamin C–rich foods had less wrinkling and dryness.

Chocolate may give skin a healthier appearance. Cocoa butter applied to the skin can help diminish stretch marks. According to one intriguing study, women who drank high-flavanol cocoa beverages had decreased roughness and scaling of the skin.

Apples, beans, tea, olive oil, vegetables, and dried plums. A study published in the *Journal of the American College of Nutrition* described promising findings for people who live in high-sun-exposure areas. Elderly men and women (of various ethnicities) had less skin wrinkling with a higher intake of vegetables, olive oil, legumes, apples, tea, and dried plums.

Optimal Life Supplements

A *multivitamin* with adequate levels of vitamins A, C, and E is worth adding to your daily diet, especially if you don't get enough of these nutrients from the food you eat and spend a lot of time in the sun. And using a topical vitamin C cream may help protect skin cells from free radical damage associated with the effects of aging.

Feeding the Fire!

Saturated fat in butter and in other fatty animal products and trans fats found in margarines have been associated with increased wrinkling in the elderly.

BEAUTIFUL SKIN MENU PLAN

Day 1

Breakfast (425)
1 cup flaxseed cereal flakes (190)
1 cup skim milk (90)
1 kiwi (60)
½ cup orange juice (60)
1 teaspoon honey (25)
1 cup green tea

Lunch (430)
1 serving *Roasted Vegetable and Sweet Swiss Panini* (250)
(page 333)
6 whole grain crackers (130)
1 cup strawberries (50)
1½ cups water with lemon

Midday Snack (220)
1 serving *Chilean Fruit Guacamole* (100) (page 259)
12 fat-free corn chips (120)
1½ cups sparkling water with lime

Dinner (700)
4 ounces rotisserie chicken (220)
1 cup steamed Brussels sprouts (60)
1 serving *Polenta Pizza* (180) (page 329)
2 cups spinach salad with assorted veggies and citrus dressing (120)
5 ounces red wine (optional) (120)

Evening Snack (240)
1 cup carrot sticks (50)
2 tablespoons hummus (60)
1 serving *Apple-Soy Chai Latte* (130) (page 254)

———————

Day 2

Breakfast (350)
1 serving *Soufflé Omelet with Balsamic Strawberries* (160) (page 345)
4 to 5 dried plums (100)
1 cup skim milk (90)

Lunch (440)
1 serving *Blackberry Smoothie* (320) (page 258)
1 serving *Avocado-Fennel Citrus Salad* (120) (page 285)

Midday Snack (290)
1 serving *Rosemary Nuts* (290) (page 269)
1 cup green tea

Dinner (688)
1 serving *Cocoa-Encrusted Salmon with Blueberries* (270)
(page 330)
2 servings *Roasted Autumn Vegetables in Sherry Sauce* (228)
(page 360)
1 whole grain roll (100)
1 cup skim milk (90)

Evening Snack (240)
. 1 serving *Beanie-Greenie Brownies* (110) (page 309)
1 serving *Apple-Soy Chai Latte* (130) (page 254)

Day 3

Breakfast (453)
1 serving *Triple-Grain Georgia Pecan Pancakes* (188) (page 346)
½ cup hash browns (120)
½ cup diced mango (55)
1 cup skim milk (90)

Lunch (440)
1 serving *Tropical Fruit and Shrimp Gazpacho* (80) (page 279)
1 serving *Raw Kale Salad with Lemon-Honey Vinaigrette* (260)
(page 296)
1 whole grain roll (100)
1½ cups water with lemon

Midday Snack (130)
1 serving *Strawberry-Papaya Smoothie* (130) (page 255)

Dinner (546)
1 serving *Chicken Thighs with Red Wine, Dried Plums, and
Garlic* (310) (page 323)

1 serving *Sicilian Broccoli Salad* (200) (page 291)
1 serving *Watermelon Soda* (36) (page 253)

Evening Snack (480)
1 serving *Summer Fruits Pie* (390) (page 315)
1 cup skim milk (90)

Dr. Gary Jay Barsky's Tips for Healthy Skin

Gary Jay Barsky, MD, is a Harvard-trained physician and board-certified dermatologist who practices in the Chicago metropolitan area. He is also certified through the American Board of Cosmetic Surgery and the American Board of Laser Surgery. Visit www.drbarsky.com.

Great nutrition is one essential part of the healthy-skin equation. Try to incorporate as many of these great suggestions into your daily activities as you can:

1. Don't smoke!
2. Avoid overexposure to the sun and avoid tanning beds. Use artificial tanning creams instead.
3. Stop facial exercises.
4. Wear protective clothing including wide-brimmed hats and long sleeves if you are outdoors for long periods during the day.
5. Apply a broad-spectrum sunscreen that offers UVA and UVB protection with a sun protection factor (SPF) of 15 or higher. Use a sunscreen with zinc and titanium.
6. Regular exercise promotes good blood flow and greater delivery of oxygen to the skin.
7. Use topical vitamin C creams to help reduce free radicals and fine lines and improve the skin's appearance.
8. Many people are zinc deficient, but don't know it. Topical ointments with zinc oxide help protect the skin.

9. Soy milk has natural estrogens in the right amounts and promotes healing. Estrogen helps keep the face firm.

ECZEMA

"Erupting Skin"

Did you know... *over 15 million people in the United States have
some form of eczema?*

Optimal Food/Nutrient Highlights

Fatty fish, walnuts, soybeans, flaxseed oil, canola oil, probiotics.

What Is Eczema?

Eczema refers to a group of noncontagious skin conditions. The
most common form of eczema is atopic dermatitis, which affects 10
to 20 percent of the world population. Eczema is an inflammatory
response to substances that cause irritation to the skin. In most
cases, eczema can be managed well with treatment and the avoidance of triggers.

What Causes It?

Although eczema's cause is unknown, it appears to be an abnormal
response of the body's immune system. Some forms of eczema
can be triggered by substances that come in contact with the skin,
such as soaps, cosmetics, clothing, detergents, jewelry, or sweat.

Environmental allergens (substances that cause allergic reactions) may also cause outbreaks. Changes in temperature or humidity, or even psychological stress, may lead to outbreaks. If your mother or a sibling has eczema, you're probably at increased risk of developing it yourself.

Optimal Life Foods

Fatty fish, walnuts, soybeans, flaxseed oil, and canola oil. According to a recent study of 5,000 children, those who consumed fish early on in life were 24 percent less likely to develop eczema in childhood.

Optimal Life Supplements

Gamma-linolenic acid (GLA). Studies on GLA supplements such as evening primrose oil and borage oil have returned mixed results. In some older studies, GLA was shown to decrease inflammation, but in recent years, GLA has not shown great clinical success. Nevertheless, evening primrose oil has been approved for use in treating atopic dermatitis in countries outside of the United States.

Probiotics, a variety of friendly bacteria known to promote digestion and a healthy immune system, have shown promise for reducing or preventing atopic eczema/dermatitis in children. Infants benefit when moms take probiotics during pregnancy and breastfeeding. Probiotics may stabilize the intestinal barrier function and decrease gastrointestinal symptoms in children with atopic dermatitis.

Aloe, chamomile, licorice, and witch hazel, prepared in topical formulas, have shown promise in reducing symptoms of eczema.

Fish oil contains omega-3 fats, which help reduce inflammatory skin disorders.

Caution! *Purchase dietary supplements that are free of common allergens such as dairy, wheat, eggs, nuts, seafood, and artificial food additives, preservatives, and colorings.*

Feeding the Fire!

There's a good deal of confusion about when a parent should introduce common allergenic foods into her child's diet. Although researchers have found that children who are breast-fed for up to the first two years of life have the lowest risk of eczema, allergies, and asthma, experts continue to disagree over the basics. My clinical experience is mixed, as well. As a general rule, however, I always advise moms to breast-feed for as long as possible and not to rush foods into their children's diets.

Allergenic foods most often include eggs, dairy, wheat, nuts, shellfish, tomatoes, and citrus.

ECZEMA-RELIEF MENU PLAN

Day 1

Breakfast (470)
1 serving *Creamy Cherry Oatmeal* (210) (substitute soy milk
for the 2% milk—calories will be slightly less depending on
brand; page 350)
1 cup light soy milk (110)
1 kiwi (50)

½ cup Concord grape juice (70)
1 teaspoon honey (25)
1 cup green tea

Lunch (457)
1 serving *Winter White Bean Chili* (257) (page 282)
6 gluten-free rice crackers (130)
1 cup raspberries (70)
1½ cups water

Midday Snack (220)
1 serving *Chilean Fruit Guacamole* (100) (page 259)
12 fat-free corn chips (120)
1½ cups sparkling water

Dinner (730)
4 ounces rotisserie chicken (220)
1 cup steamed broccoli florets (50)
1 serving *Polenta Pizza* (180) (page 329)
1 serving *Barley Salad with Edamame* (160) (page 287)
5 ounces red wine (optional) (120)

Evening Snack (205)
½ cup carrot sticks (25)
2 tablespoons hummus (50)
1 serving *Apple-Soy Chai Latte* (130) (page 254)

Day 2

Breakfast (450)
1 serving *Capp-oat-ccino Delight* (340) (page 337)
1 cup light soy milk (110)

Lunch (546)
1 serving *Quick Pumpkin Smoothie* (230) (substitute soy yogurt
for the fat-free yogurt; page 256)
1 serving *Bean-Corn Salad* (120) (page 290)
1 serving *Asian Satay Skewers with Black Bean Sauce* (196)
(page 263)
1½ cups water

Midday Snack (240)
1 serving *Cherry–Chai Spice Granola* (240) (page 348)
1 cup green tea

Dinner (670)
1 serving *Mediterranean Grilled Mackerel or Bluefish* (250)
(leave out the lemon juice; page 321)
1 serving *Asparagus-Carrot Rolls* (210) (page 361)
1 gluten-free roll (100)
1 cup light soy milk (110)

Evening Snack (165)
1 serving *Poached Pears* (165) (page 307)
1 cup decaffeinated green tea

Day 3

Breakfast (580)
3 gluten-free pancakes made with ground flaxseeds (240)
½ cup hash browns (120)
1 cup diced mango (110)
1 cup light soy milk (110)

Lunch (430)
1 serving *Winter Squash Soup with Roasted Seeds* (70) (page 277)
1 serving *Raw Kale Salad with Lemon-Honey Vinaigrette* (260)
(substitute 3 tablespoons of balsamic vinegar and olive oil
blend for the lemon juice; page 296)
1 gluten-free roll (100)
1½ cups water

Midday Snack (130)
1 serving *Apple-Soy Chai Latte* (130) (page 254)

Dinner (646)
1 serving *Chicken Thighs with Red Wine, Dried Plums, and
Garlic* (310) (page 323)
1 serving *Sicilian Broccoli Salad* (200) (page 291)
½ cup brown rice (100)
1 serving *Watermelon Soda* (36) (page 253)

Evening Snack (150)
1 serving *Pan-Cooked Apples and Pears in Grape Juice* (150)
(page 313)
1 cup decaffeinated green tea

Dr. Barsky's Tips

1. For pregnant and lactating women: Take a multivitamin with
   antioxidants during pregnancy. A study of 2,000 women found
   that those who had adequate antioxidant intake during pregnancy had a lower risk of their children developing eczema during early childhood.
2. Keep the affected areas clean and moist. Apply lotions with
   clean, dry hands.
3. Avoid alcohol-based hand sanitizers and gels.

4. Wear clothes made of soft fabrics like cotton, and avoid scatchy fabrics like wool. Wash all new clothing before wearing it.

5. Psychological and emotional stress may be a contributing factor. Discover a relaxation method that suits you and practice it on a regular basis.

6. Avoid coffee and spicy foods.

7. Take a vitamin D_3 supplement.

8. Avoid exposure to tobacco smoke and chemicals such as paint and bleach.

9. Air-conditioning and extremes in temperature can also aggravate excema.

PSORIASIS

Getting Under Your Skin

Did you know..._psoriasis is a risk factor for cardiovascular disease?_

Optimal Food/Nutrient Highlights

Vegetarian and diets including fatty fish, whey, CoQ$_{10}$, and selenium.

What Is Psoriasis?

Psoriasis, which affects more than 5 million American adults, is one of the most difficult skin disorders to treat. The cells multiply much more quickly than normal skin cells, and when they die, they're responsible for the appearance of red thickened plaques with white scales on the skin. Psoriasis most often appears on the knees, elbows, scalp, torso, palms, and soles of the feet.

What Causes It?

Although science has yet to find the cause of this troubling condition, psoriasis has been linked to emotional stress, trauma to the skin, streptococcal infection, immune system abnormality, and drug reactions to ibuprofen and the antimalarial medication chloroquine. Thirty percent of sufferers have a family history of it. Fortunately, in one-third of patients, the symptoms disappear by themselves.

Optimal Life Foods

Vegetarian diets and diets including fatty fish have been shown to improve psoriasis symptoms. Flaxseed, flaxseed oil, walnuts, and canola oil are a few ways for those vegetarians who don't eat fish to get in their omega-3 fats.

Optimal Life Supplements

CoQ$_{10}$, vitamin E, and selenium supplements led to significant improvement in the red plaque otherwise known as "lesions" compared with a placebo.

When used topically, *vitamins D and B$_{12}$, avocado, and fish oil* may help relieve skin irritation.

Whey. A small study showed significant improvement in those subjects who took a whey supplement versus a placebo.

Feeding the Fire!

Diabetes, obesity, metabolic syndrome, and hypertension have all been associated with a higher occurrence of psoriasis. These conditions suggest that weight loss through a controlled-calorie diet and exercise program is in order. A gluten-free diet may also be beneficial to those with a gluten sensitivity that spurs on psoriasis.

PSORIASIS-FIGHTING MENU PLAN

Day 1

Breakfast (445)
1 serving *Creamy Cherry Oatmeal* (210) (use gluten-free oats; page 350)
1 cup skim milk (90)
1 kiwi (50)
½ cup Concord grape juice (70)
1 teaspoon honey (25)
1 cup green tea

Lunch (457)
1 serving *Winter White Bean Chili* (257) (page 282)
6 gluten-free rice crackers (130)
1 cup raspberries (70)
1½ cups water with lemon

Midday Snack (220)
1 serving *Chilean Fruit Guacamole* (100) (page 259)
12 fat-free corn chips (120)
1½ cups sparkling water with lime

Dinner (690)

4 ounces rotisserie chicken (220)

1 cup steamed broccoli florets (50)

½ cup brown rice (100)

1 serving *Avocado-Fennel Citrus Salad* (120) (page 285)

½ cup Concord grape juice (70)

1 serving *Spicy Biscotti* (130) (page 311)

Evening Snack (205)

½ cup carrot sticks (25)

2 tablespoons hummus (50)

1 serving *Apple-Soy Chai Latte* (130) (page 254)

Day 2

Breakfast (490)

1 serving *Chef Wiley's Granola* (290) (use gluten-free oats; page 351)

5 dried plums (110)

1 cup skim milk (90)

Lunch (445)

1 serving *Apple-Soy Chai Latte* (130) (page 254)

1 serving *Curried Chickpeas and Kale* (150) (page 370)

1 serving *Poached Pears* (165) (page 307)

1½ cups water with lemon

Midday Snack (195)

¼ cup dry-roasted soy nuts (195)

1 cup green tea

Dinner (650)
1 serving *Mediterranean Grilled Mackerel or Bluefish* (250)
(page 321)
1 serving *Asparagus-Carrot Rolls* (210) (page 361)
1 gluten-free roll (100)
1 cup skim milk (90)

Evening Snack (140)
1 serving *Christine's Baked Custard* (140) (page 308)
1 cup decaffeinated green tea

Day 3

Breakfast (480)
1 serving *Soufflé Omelet with Balsamic Strawberries* (160)
(page 345)
½ cup hash browns (120)
1 cup diced mango (110)
1 cup skim milk (90)

Lunch (560)
1 serving *Winter Squash Soup with Roasted Seeds* (70) (page 277)
1 serving *Raw Kale Salad with Lemon-Honey Vinaigrette* (260)
(page 296)
1 serving *Quick Pumpkin Smoothie* (230) (page 256)

Midday Snack (130)
1 serving *Apple-Soy Chai Latte* (130) (page 254)

Dinner (686)
1 serving *Irish Poached Salmon* (350) (page 320)
1 serving *Sicilian Broccoli Salad* (200) (page 291)

½ cup brown rice (100)
1 serving *Watermelon Soda* (36) (page 253)

Evening Snack (150)
1 serving *Raspberry Salsa* (30) (page 299)
12 fat free corn chips (120)
1 cup decaffeinated green tea

Dr. Barsky's Tips

1. Practice relaxation and stress-management techniques.
2. Don't smoke.
3. Reduce alcohol consumption.
4. Consult a dermatologist for the kinds of lotions and creams that will help to maintain moist skin.
5. Take care of skin infections as soon as they occur.
6. Dandruff is a cousin of psoriasis: Avoid hot beverages, very hot showers, irritating shampoos, and hair dryers.

ACNE

Face It—It's Coming to a Head

Did you know...*nearly 95 percent of the population has experienced acne at least one time in their lives?*

Optimal Food/Nutrient Highlights

Vitamin A–, vitamin C–, and zinc-rich foods, whole wheat, cumin, coriander, fennel, fatty fish, flaxseed, yogurt, sauerkraut.

What Is Acne?

Acne vulgaris is the scientific term for what we normally call clogged pores that result in pimples, blackheads, whiteheads, or nodules that form on various places on the body. Acne results from the overproduction of sebum, a waxy substance that lubricates the skin. Sebum plugs up hair follicles, causing bacteria growth.

Although acne is most often thought of as a teenage curse, adults well into their forties can be haunted by flare-ups (as I well know!) and it can be the source of much physical and emotional scarring.

ACNE SPEAK

Comedo: A plugged follicle.

Blackhead: A blemish that has a dark and open center.

Whitehead: A blemish that bulges under the skin and has no opening.

Pimple: A whitehead that ruptures.

Papule: A small, solid, slightly elevated lesion.

Pustule: A dome-shaped lesion containing pus.

Macule: A red spot left on the skin from a healed lesion.

Nodule: A solid, dome-shaped lesion. Often attributed to "scarring" acne and more resistant to treatment.

Cyst: A saclike lesion, larger than a pustule, containing pus and liquid. Cysts and nodules together are called nodulocystic acne.

What Causes It?

Hormonal changes that occur during adolescence, pregnancy, or starting or stopping birth control medication probably play a role in acne. There may also be a genetic link; if your folks had it at one time, there is a high likelihood that you may be visited by it, too. Sorry, kids! Although dirty skin does not cause acne, sensitivity to make-up, creams, and even some medications may cause outbreaks.

Dr. Barsky recommends a multistep hygiene regime: Wash, but do not scrub, as often necessary as to keep the area clean. Shampoo hair regularly. Keep long hair off the face and shoulders. When shaving, use a fresh blade to minimize the chance of spreading the infection; take care to avoid nicking pimples. If you have to wear makeup, use only the hypoallergenic, fragrance-free kind, and avoid applying cosmetics to acne-prone areas. Don't pop, pick, scratch, or squeeze your pimples. This may cause infection or scarring.

ACNE MYTH BUSTERS

Myth #1: Chocolate and greasy foods cause acne. No evidence to date. However, the skin is a reflection of overall health, and too much chocolate and greasy food does not serve you or your skin well!

Myth #2: Stress causes acne. I know I seem to get more breakouts when I'm feeling stressed. However, no evidence to date has linked stress to acne. Paradoxically, some studies have shown that those who perceive they have stress tend to have *more* acne, or that stress can make acne worse.

Optimal Life Foods

> *Carmina McGee, MS, RD, is a registered dietitian, a licensed aesthetician, and an expert on nutritional approaches to fighting acne. I have included her top food recommendations along with mine in this section.*

Vitamin A heavies such as carrots, broccoli, tomatoes, sweet potatoes, mangoes, guavas, kale, pumpkins, and spinach are essential for healthy skin and critical for those with acne. Six to nine servings of fruits and vegetables a day will help keep acne away. These same vegetables also support your liver's detoxification ability.

Vitamin C–rich foods like peppers, strawberries, kiwis, and citrus fruits quench inflammation and improve healing of wounds caused by acne lesions.

Zinc is a key mineral for acne control. Whole grains, nuts, poultry, and lean red meats are great ways to get zinc into your body.

Whole wheat. Derivatives of wheat kernels called *puroindolines* were found to be effective in killing staphylococcal bacteria associated with acne.

Cumin, coriander, and fennel. Try this acne home remedy from India: Combine a half teaspoon each of cumin, coriander, and whole fennel seeds in a tea ball and steep in hot water for ten minutes. Strain and drink the tea after breakfast, lunch, and dinner.

Salmon, tuna, mackerel, and sardines are just a few examples of fish rich in omega-3 fats that help douse the flames of inflammation.

Flaxseed, canola, walnuts, soy, and hempseed are good vegetarian sources of the omega-3 fat alpha-linolenic acid.

Yogurt, sauerkraut, kimchi, and unpasteurized miso are all excellent sources of friendly bacteria, also known as probiotics.

Optimal Life Supplements

I had bad acne during my teen years. I was working at a health food store at the time and a customer recommended three supplements that he felt would help. Did they ever! I really scoured the scientific literature for a reason why this combo worked but came up empty-handed. The upside is that I couldn't find a downside to taking the combo either, so it might be worth a try:

- *Hyland's NuAge Tissue D Acne.* This formula contains four homeopathic tissue salts: Kali Muriaticum 6X HPUS, Kali Sulphuricum 3X HPUS, Calcarea Sulphurica 3X HPUS, and Silica 12X HPUS. Take as directed (four tablets dissolved under the tongue, three times per day). Don't worry—the tablets are really small!
- *Aloe vera gel.* One to two ounces a day—be careful! Aloe can have a laxative effect.
- *Nutritional yeast.* One to two tablespoons per day. This one isn't so far-fetched when you think about it. Nutritional yeast is loaded with B vitamins and other nutrients that are good for the skin and have been favorably reviewed in science journals.

Nicotinamide, a form of the B vitamin niacin, may reduce inflammatory lesions associated with both acne vulgaris and rosacea.

Vitamin B_6 aids in the metabolism of hormones that can spur on acne.

Fish oil. A small study showed improvement of acne lesions for those subjects who consumed fish oil supplements.

Topical application of vitamins A, C, E, and B_3 may improve acne lesions.

Zinc may help contribute to reducing inflammation and helps heal damaged skin caused by acne.

Vitamin A reduces sebum and keratin production.

Caution! *Taking megadoses of vitamin A can cause headaches, fatigue, muscle and joint pain, and other side effects.*

Vitamin D is great for overall skin health.

Feeding the Fire!

Most dermatologists advocate an overall healthy diet for promoting healthy skin, and many feel that there isn't enough evidence to single out any one acne-causing food. Several "alternative" doctors outside of the mainstream contend that all acne is the result of an inflammatory process (regardless of whether the acne you have is considered "inflammatory" or not). I sit squarely in the camp of tailored nutrition. Cause and effect can be a pretty powerful thing, so if you already know that you break out when you eat certain foods, then who cares what "research" says, right? Do what's right for *you*! But if you're not quite sure what foods may be problematic, consider the following list of potential offenders. Try eliminating them, one at a time, from your diet for a week and see if it makes a difference. If not, then celebrate and welcome back that food into your diet (but not with reckless abandon!).

Dairy. One study found a correlation between dairy consumption and acne in teenage boys. Unfortunately, this study was based on a self-reported questionnaire and did not exclude other possible reasons for acne. If you do decide to eliminate dairy from your diet, include adequate dietary sources of calcium. Dairy is also known to increase insulin-like growth factor (IGF-1), a hormone that has been implicated in increasing sebum.

Calories. Caloric restriction has been shown to help control the production of IGF-1. However, reduce calories only if you are overweight.

A low-glycemic-load diet. A high-glycemic-load diet and dairy together have been associated with increasing IGF-1. A small study evaluated the effects of either a high- or a low-glycemic-load diet on acne. Both the control and intervention groups had lesion reductions, but the groups assigned to a low-glycemic-load diet had the greatest reductions in acne lesions. A healthy version of a low-glycemic-load diet entails:

- Moderate consumption of whole grains and fruits.
- Lower consumption of starchy foods such as potatoes, rice, and breads and of refined-carbohydrate foods like sugary drinks and sweet bakery goods.
- Increased consumption of nonstarchy vegetables, nuts, beans, and lean proteins.

Carmina McGee's Tips for Managing Acne

1. Go easy on milk, particularly if you are dairy-sensitive, and choose organic to keep hormones from the outside to a minimum.
2. If you have been on antibiotic treatment, once it is over, take probiotics on a daily basis to restore and rebalance the intestinal tract. Probiotics will also help support your immune system to fight acne-causing bacteria.
3. Find moments throughout the day to mellow out. Managing stress will help manage your acne.
4. When you look in the mirror, focus on the beauty and perfection you are as a human being; be kind and gentle to yourself. Don't let a little acne define who you are or how you think of yourself.

ACNE-FIGHTING MENU PLAN

I've left some dairy in this menu plan. I haven't seen many patients respond to the complete elimination of dairy; however, if you don't see improvement in your skin by following our recommendations for a week or so, try eliminating dairy as "plan B."

Day 1

Breakfast (380)
1 cup flaxseed cereal flakes (190)
1 cup almond milk (110)
½ cup guava (55)
1 teaspoon honey (25)
1 cup green tea

Lunch (420)
1 serving *Roasted Vegetable and Sweet Swiss Panini* (250) (the cheese can be left off if you like; page 333)
6 whole wheat crackers (120)
1 cup strawberries (50)
1½ cups water with lemon

Midday Snack (440)
1 serving *Sardine Salad / Dip* (320) (page 265)
6 whole wheat crackers (120)
1½ cups sparkling water with lime

Dinner (590)
4 ounces rotisserie chicken (220)

1 serving *Fingerling Potatoes with Asparagus* (250) (page 363)

2 cups spinach salad with assorted veggies and citrus dressing (120)

1 cup decaffeinated green tea

Evening Snack (205)

½ cup carrot sticks (25)

2 tablespoons hummus (50)

1 serving *Apple-Soy Chai Latte* (130) (page 254)

Day 2

Breakfast (540)

1 serving *Zucchini-Cranberry Muffins* (190) (page 339)

1 serving *Cherry–Chai Spice Granola* (240) (page 348)

1 cup light soy milk (110)

Lunch (540)

1 serving *Blackberry Smoothie* (320) (page 258)

1 serving *Avocado-Fennel Citrus Salad* (120) (page 285)

1 whole wheat roll (100)

Midday Snack (290)

1 serving *Rosemary Nuts* (290) (page 269)

1 cup green tea

Dinner (594)

1 serving *Cocoa-Encrusted Salmon with Blueberries* (270) (page 330)

1 serving *Roasted Autumn Vegetables in Sherry Sauce* (114) (page 360)

1 whole grain roll (100)
1 cup almond milk (110)

Evening Snack (110)
1 serving *Beanie-Greenie Brownies* (110) (page 309)
1 cup decaffeinated green tea

Day 3

Breakfast (493)
1 serving *Triple-Grain Georgia Pecan Pancakes* (188)
(page 346)
1 turkey sausage link (140)
½ cup diced mango (55)
1 cup light soy milk (110)

Lunch (440)
1 serving *Tropical Fruit and Shrimp Gazpacho* (80)
(page 279)
1 serving *Raw Kale Salad with Lemon-Honey Vinaigrette* (260)
(page 296)
1 whole grain roll (100)
1½ cups water with lemon

Midday Snack (130)
1 serving *Strawberry-Papaya Smoothie* (130) (page 255)

Dinner (736)
1 serving *Chicken Thighs with Red Wine, Dried Plums, and
Garlic* (310) (page 323)
1 serving *Asparagus-Sesame Stir-Fry* (100) (page 362)

1 serving *Wild Mushroom Ris-oat-to* (290) (page 357)

1 serving *Watermelon Soda* (36) (page 253)

Evening Snack (260)

1 serving *Spicy Biscotti* (130) (page 311)

1 serving *Apple-Soy Chai Latte* (130) (page 254)

PART 2

GO WITH THE FLOW

COLD FEET (AND HANDS)

When the Shoe Drops . . .

Did you know ... *the* Oxford English Dictionary *attributes the early use of the term* cold feet *to writer and poet Stephen Crane? In his book* Maggie: A Girl of the Streets, *published in the late 1800s, Crane wrote, "I knew this was the way it would be. They got cold feet." Other sources suggest that the term was associated with decisions made (or not made) under the duress of literally having cold feet from the lack of proper footwear. It was thought that the absence of footwear would make one more hesitant and cautious.*

Optimal Food/Nutrient Highlights

Arginine-rich foods, berries, vegetables, spices, tea, wine, chocolate, chile peppers, omega-3 fats.

What Causes Cold Feet and Hands?

Cold feet and hands are often due to poor circulation or other underlying medical disorders that affect the nervous system.

Most everyone experiences cold feet or cold hands at one time or another, especially when the weather turns cooler. But for some, the condition is not limited to the change of the seasons; it can be a sign of a more serious health problem. The most common cause of cold feet and hands is poor circulation, especially in the elderly.

Smoking causes blood vessels to constrict.

Iron deficiencies affect one in five pregnant women, and iron helps red blood cells carry oxygen.

Peripheral neuropathy results from damage to the nerves in the vessels that supply blood to the feet and hands.

Raynaud's phenomenon is a disorder of the small blood vessels that feed the skin. Feet and hands that turn blue, swell, or lose sensation could be signs of Raynaud's phenomenon.

Hypothyroidism is a condition resulting from an underactive thyroid gland.

Peripheral vascular disease, a condition that involves narrowing of the arteries, restricts blood flow to the extremities and other parts of the body.

Medications such as beta-blockers, migraine relievers, and hormone replacement therapy and chemotherapy agents may cause blood vessels to narrow.

Carpal tunnel syndrome is a condition where the median nerve becomes compressed at the wrist, resulting in pain, weakness, numbness, and a cold sensation in the hand, wrist, and arm.

Working with vibrating machinery, typing, or playing piano excessively may cause trauma or injury to feet or hands.

Frostbite causes damage to skin and nerve endings in the extremities.

Optimal Life Foods

Arginine-rich foods. Arginine is an amino acid that helps produce nitric oxide in the body. Nitric oxide helps to expand the diameter of the lumen of the vessels that run throughout the circulatory system, allowing more blood to flow through. Foods rich in arginine include peanuts, almonds, walnuts, Brazil nuts, soybeans, dairy, pork, beef, chicken, turkey, oats, wheat, barley, chickpeas, salmon, tuna, and mackerel.

Fruits, vegetables, herbs, and spices. A diet of fruits and vegetables, particularly those rich in antioxidant compounds called flavonoids, has been shown to improve the health of blood vessels. Fruits and vegetables of optimal benefit include Concord grapes, pomegranates, raspberries, strawberries, cranberries, cherries, apples, kale, broccoli, parsley, celery, onions, and chiles. The herb thyme and cinnamon are also beneficial.

Tea (especially green tea), wine, and chocolate possess catechins, tannins, flavonoids, and other polyphenolic compounds that encourage nitric oxide formation in cells to improve circulation. Cocoa flavanols help promote vasodilation (expansion of the blood vessels), which promotes good circulation. Ingesting cocoa was found to decrease the stickiness of blood platelets for up to two hours after consumption.

Chile peppers contain a substance called capsaicin known to enhance circulation. Sprinkling a little cayenne pepper in your shoes and gloves helps keep toes and fingers toasty.

Optimal Life Supplements

Butcher's broom is an herb that, according to a German study of 166 women, has proved to be a safe and effective treatment for chronic venous insufficiency (CVI), a state of diminished blood flow through the veins of the leg.

Horse chestnut is another herb that is a safe alternative for treating CVI.

Fish oil supplements improved symptoms of Raynaud's phenomenon in one small study. Researchers from Albany Medical College in New York found that those subjects who took fish oil supplements were symptom-free at the end of the three-month study. Omega-3 fats reduced painful spasms that caused decreased blood flow to both toes and fingers.

Grape seeds contain a variety of polyphenols that help protect blood vessels from the damage of inflammation and help them retain their flexibility. Proanthocyanidins are a group of compounds found in grapes that help improve blood circulation by strengthening capillaries, arteries, and veins. You may obtain the grape seeds in the form of grape seed extract.

Ginseng contains plant chemicals called saponins, which have been shown to relax blood vessels, thus enhancing blood flow.

Feeding the Fire!

Alcohol dilates blood vessels, which initially makes you feel warm; yet after a while, the dilated vessels cause the body to throw off heat.

Caffeine consumed in excessive amounts can constrict blood vessels. Limit yourself to no more than twenty-four ounces of caffeinated coffee per day. This is the eqivalent of three cups of coffee.

A *diet high in saturated and trans fats* can lead to clogging of the arteries.

TOASTY FEET AND HANDS MENU PLAN

Day 1

Breakfast (425)
1 serving *Cherry–Chai Spice Granola* (240) (page 348)
1 cup skim milk (90)
½ cup Concord grape juice (70)
1 teaspoon honey (25)
1 cup green tea

Lunch (460)
1 serving *Roasted Vegetable and Sweet Swiss Panini* (250) (page 333)
1 ounce almonds (160)
1 cup strawberries (50)
1½ cups water with lemon

Midday Snack (220)
1 serving *Chilean Fruit Guacamole* (100) (page 259)

12 fat-free corn chips (120)

1½ cups sparkling water with lime

Dinner (750)

1 serving *Grilled Chicken Salad with Pomegranate Vinaigrette and Mango Gelée Garnish* (300) (page 324)

1 serving *Roasted Root Vegetables* (240) (page 365)

1 serving *Sharon's Moroccan Couscous* (210) (page 359)

1 cup decaffeinated green tea

Evening Snack (205)

½ cup carrot sticks (25)

2 tablespoons hummus (50)

1 serving *Apple-Soy Chai Latte* (130) (page 254)

Day 2

Breakfast (510)

1 serving *Soufflé Omelet with Balsamic Strawberries* (160) (page 345)

1 whole grain bagel (230)

1 serving *Fruit and Walnut Jam Conserve* (30) (page 302)

1 cup skim milk (90)

Lunch (440)

1 serving *Blackberry Smoothie* (320) (page 258)

1 serving *Avocado-Fennel Citrus Salad* (120) (page 285)

Midday Snack (290)

1 serving *Rosemary Nuts* (290) (page 269)

1 cup green tea

Dinner (610)
1 serving *Cocoa-Encrusted Salmon with Blueberries* (270)
(page 330)
1 serving *Curried Chickpeas and Kale* (150) (page 370)
1 whole grain roll (100)
1 cup skim milk (90)

Evening Snack (216)
1 serving *Crumb-Topped Georgia Pecan and Cherry Cereal
Bars* (216) (page 341)
1 cup decaffeinated green tea

Day 3

Breakfast (428)
1 serving *Triple-Grain Georgia Pecan Pancakes* (188) (page 346)
1 serving *Fruit and Walnut Jam Conserve* (30) (page 302)
½ cup hash browns (120)
1 cup skim milk (90)

Lunch (440)
1 serving *Tropical Fruit and Shrimp Gazpacho* (80) (page 279)
1 serving *Raw Kale Salad with Lemon-Honey Vinaigrette* (260)
(page 296)
1 whole grain roll (100)
1½ cups water with lemon

Midday Snack (130)
1 serving *Strawberry-Papaya Smoothie* (130) (page 255)

Dinner (736)
1 serving *Chicken Thighs with Red Wine, Dried Plums, and
Garlic* (310) (page 323)

1 serving *Warm Goat Cheese Salad with Hazelnuts and Raspberries* (390) (page 295)
1 serving *Watermelon Soda* (36) (page 253)

Evening Snack (298)
1 serving *Chile-Honey Almond Chicken Kebabs* (261) (page 266)
1 cup skim milk (90)

Dave's Tips

1. Don't smoke; get physical; and lose weight. These three choices alone have the most significant impact on circulation.
2. Eat fish at least twice a week. Omega-3 fats help improve circulation.
3. Eat more vegetables such as peppers, onions, and garlic and fruits such as strawberries, raspberries, blueberries, and grapes, which contain anti-inflammatory properties.

LEG CRAMPS

That's Lame!

Did you know... *there are many theories on how the term* charley horse *came to be? One popular story is that there was a lame horse named Charley who worked at the Chicago White Sox ballpark (Comiskey Park). After that, lame horses were referred to as Charley. Another story dates back to the 1880s, when pitcher Charley "Old Hoss" Radbourne suffered from a cramp in his leg during a game.*

Optimal Food/Nutrient Highlights

Carb-laden foods, sodium, calcium, potassium, magnesium, vitamin E.

What Are Leg Cramps?

Leg cramps are involuntary and sustained contractions of one or more muscles that result in pain and immobility. Such cramps are extremely common—at least 95 percent of us experience cramping at some point. Leg cramps become increasingly frequent as we age.

What Causes Them?

Muscles tighten for a variety of reasons, such as lack of fluids, injury, muscle strain, or staying in the same position for a long period of time. Blood-circulation problems or pressure on the nerves in the spine can also cause cramplike pains in your legs.

Some common causes of night leg cramps include muscle overexertion, prolonged sitting, dehydration, pregnancy, diabetes, decreased potassium levels, neuromuscular disorders (such as Parkinson's disease and other underlying diseases), side effects of certain medications, alcohol use, and malnutrition.

Optimal Life Foods

Carbohydrates. Athletes, especially, should have adequate carbohydrate intake to prevent premature muscle fatigue during exercise. Sources of healthy carbohydrates include fruits, vegetables, and whole grains.

Sodium. Salt contains the mineral sodium and can be found in a variety of foods and in sports drinks. Sodium, along with other minerals discussed below (known as electrolytes), can help prevent heat cramping. If you see salt on your skin after the sweat dries, then you may need to increase salty foods before exercise. However, most Americans get more than enough sodium in their diets.

Calcium. When you experience leg cramps, another factor to consider is your calcium intake. Calcium plays an essential role in muscle contractions, so you should include some milk, yogurt, or another calcium-rich food in your diet every day.

Potassium-containing foods. Strawberries, papaya, dried plums, cantaloupe, bananas, raisins, mangoes, kiwis, oranges, pears, peaches, watermelon, apples, pineapple, tomatoes, potatoes, sweet potatoes, avocados, asparagus, pumpkin, mushrooms, Brussels sprouts, green beans, carrots, broccoli.

Magnesium. Include foods like oatmeal, almonds, halibut, wheat bran, pumpkin seeds, barley, buckwheat flour, low-fat vanilla yogurt, trail mix, chickpeas, lima beans, soybeans, and spinach.

Optimal Life Supplements

Magnesium. An animal study showed that rats that ate a magnesium-deficient diet were more susceptible to muscle cramps. Their pain was promptly relieved after receiving magnesium supplements. In a human study, nighttime leg cramps were better relieved with 300 mg of magnesium supplementation when compared with a placebo.

Vitamin E might be a good choice due to its blood-thinning and vasodilating properties.

Ginkgo biloba is an herb that also provides blood-thinning effects.

Caution! *Avoid herbal diuretics that may promote dehydration and electrolyte imbalances.*

Feeding the Fire!

Excessive alcohol can contribute to dehydration.

LEG-CRAMP-RELIEF MENU PLAN

Day 1

Breakfast (515)
1 serving *Capp-oat-ccino Delight* (340) (page 337)
1 cup skim milk (90)
½ cup orange juice (60)
1 teaspoon honey (25)
1 cup green tea

Lunch (410)
1 serving *Roasted Vegetable and Sweet Swiss Panini* (250)
(page 333)
1 ounce whole grain pretzels (110)
1 cup strawberries (50)
1½ cups water with lemon

Midday Snack (220)
1 serving *Chilean Fruit Guacamole* (100) (page 259)
12 fat-free corn chips (120)
1½ cups sparkling water with lime

Dinner (690)
4 ounces rotisserie chicken strips (220)
1 serving *Nuts and Berry Fruit Salad* (350) (page 286)
5 ounces red wine (120) (optional)

Evening Snack (205)
½ cup carrot sticks (25)
2 tablespoons hummus (50)
1 cup *Apple-Soy Chai Latte* (130) (page 254)

Day 2

Breakfast (450)
1 serving *Soufflé Omelet with Balsamic Strawberries* (160)
(page 345)
1 serving *Powerhouse Dried Plum Bars* (200) (page 343)
1 cup skim milk (90)

Lunch (530)
1 serving *Quick Pumpkin Smoothie* (230) (page 256)
1 serving *Grilled Chicken Salad with Pomegranate Vinaigrette
and Mango Gelée Garnish* (300) (page 324)
1 cup green tea

Midday Snack (290)
1 serving *Rosemary Nuts* (290) (page 269)
1 cup green tea

Dinner (540)
1 serving *Dilled Salmon Cakes* (180) (page 328)
1 serving *Slow-Cooker Sweet Potatoes* (70) (page 368)

1 serving *Asparagus-Sesame Stir-Fry* (100) (page 362)
1 whole grain roll (100)
1 cup skim milk (90)

Evening Snack (220)
1 serving *Pan-Cooked Apples and Pears in Grape Juice* (150)
(page 313)
1 serving *Cheese-and-Fruit Kebabs* (70) (page 272)
1 cup decaffeinated green tea

Day 3

Breakfast (530)
1 serving *Nutty Good Millet Muffins* (240) (page 352)
2 scrambled omega-3 eggs (140)
1 cup diced papaya (60)
1 cup skim milk (90)

Lunch (440)
1 serving *Tropical Fruit and Shrimp Gazpacho* (80) (page 279)
1 serving *Raw Kale Salad with Lemon-Honey Vinaigrette* (260)
(page 296)
1 whole grain roll (100)
1½ cups water with lemon

Midday Snack (230)
1 serving *Quick Pumpkin Smoothie* (230) (page 256)

Dinner (660)
1 serving *Chicken Thighs with Red Wine, Dried Plums, and
Garlic* (310) (page 323)

1 serving *Bean-Corn Salad* (120) (page 290)
1 serving *Japanese-Style Vegetable Fried Rice* (230) (page 355)
1 cup decaffeinated green tea

Evening Snack (160)
1 serving *Cheese-and-Fruit Kebabs* (70) (page 272)
1 cup skim milk (90)

Dave's Tips

1. Straighten your leg and flex your foot toward your knee until you feel the calf muscles stretch. Try not to point your toes, as this can bring on or aggravate a cramp.
2. Don't massage your leg if you are prone to blood clots.
3. A warm bath before bedtime may also help to relax your muscles and prevent leg cramps.

PART 3

HOUSE OF PAIN

MIGRAINE HEADACHES

Famous "Brainy-Aches"

Did you know...*if you are one of the 29.5 million Americans who are bothered with migraines, you're in good company? Some famous migraine sufferers include Vincent van Gogh, Thomas Jefferson, Sigmund Freud, Elvis Presley, Elizabeth Taylor, Claude Monet, and Kareem Abdul-Jabbar.*

Optimal Food/Nutrient Highlights

Coffee, green tea, fatty fish, ginger, riboflavin, vitamin D, magnesium.

What Are Migraine Headaches?

Migraines are not your run-of-the-mill headaches. In fact, they are so incapacitating that the cost of absenteeism and diminished productivity associated with migraines in the United States is estimated to be close to $13 billion each year. The pain from a migraine is usually pulsating and occurs on one side of the head, with varying intensity from mild to severe. Nausea, vomiting, and sensitivity to light and sound are other symptoms of migraines besides pain. Some migraine sufferers experience an "aura," or a vision of bright light, but this occurs in only 15 to 20 percent of cases. Women are three times more likely to have migraines than men.

What Causes Them?

There are many theories about why migraines happen. One of the more popular theories is that the trigeminovascular system protects the brain from more serious injury like ischemia and toxins by dilating blood vessels in the brain. The downside is that this causes swelling to occur along with subsequent inflammation of those blood vessels. Activation of this system can be brought about by

- Excessive or lack of sleep.
- Excessive sun exposure.
- Inadequate blood flow to the brain.
- Dietary sensitivities.
- Hormonal changes during menses or estrogen replacement therapy. On a positive note, a study found that women who are migraine sufferers are at lower risk for estrogen-driven breast cancer due to having lower circulating estrogen.
- A reaction to medications such as antibiotics, antihyperten-

sives, histamine blockers, nonsteroidal anti-inflammatory drugs
(NSAIDs), and vasodilators.
• A reaction to physical or emotional stress.

Optimal Life Foods

Magnesium is a mineral that helps relax the nervous system.
High-magnesium foods include oatmeal, almonds, halibut, wheat
bran, pumpkin seeds, barley, buckwheat flour, chickpeas, and
spinach. Broccoli and kale are rich in magnesium.

Anti-inflammatories. Look for ways to flavor your recipes with
abundant fresh ginger; seek out omega-3 food sources such as
flaxseed, salmon, sardines, mackerel, canola, and tuna. Other anti-
inflammatory food sources include peppermint, cayenne pepper,
olive oil, and cherries. Besides having amazing anti-inflammatory
properties, tart cherries are also naturally rich in melatonin, a hormone often seen lacking in migraine sufferers.

Vitamin D. Besides sunlight, seafood such as oysters, herring, cat-
fish, cod, trout, salmon, and mackerel and fortified foods such as
dairy and soy products contain healthy amounts of vitamin D.
Mushrooms are also a best bet for vitamin D boosts that those
prone to migraines need.

Riboflavin-rich foods. Beef, especially liver, is one of the richest
sources of the B vitamin riboflavin, which helps block migraines
before they occur. Other sources include almonds, soy, mackerel,
yogurt, clams, milk, eggs, and fortified grain products.

Coffee and green tea provide caffeine, which often helps ease migraine pain. Both beverages are loaded with antioxidants that
have anti-inflammatory benefits.

Optimal Life Supplements

Riboflavin. Several studies have shown the benefits of high doses of riboflavin in the prevention of migraine headaches.

Magnesium. Low levels of magnesium are often observed in migraine and tension headache sufferers. Magnesium also controls a variety of brain chemicals known to spur on migraine headaches, including nitric oxide, which is a vasodilator. A double-blind, randomized, placebo-controlled trial found that supplementing with 600 mg of oral magnesium citrate reduced the frequency of migraine attacks by nearly 42 percent!

Feverfew. This is a popular herbal extract taken for the prevention of migraine headaches. Although a literature review of randomized, controlled feverfew trials did not find strong enough evidence for the benefits of feverfew, many of my patients who have taken the extract have reported reduced migraine pain.

CoQ$_{10}$. Deficiencies of coenzyme Q$_{10}$ have been observed in pediatric and adolescent migraine headache patients. A small study of subjects treated with CoQ$_{10}$ showed that 61 percent of them reported that they were migraine-free over 50 percent of the time during the study.

Melatonin. Six studies have established an association between melatonin and migraines. Four of these studies revealed lower levels of melatonin before, during, and after migraine onset. I advise talking to your physician or working with a registered dietitian to determine what level of melatonin supplementation may be right for you.

Olive oil and fish oil caused a reduction in the frequency, duration, and severity of migraine headaches during treatment in those patients who were taking fish oil and/or olive oil supplements.

Caution! *Avoid dietary supplements with the amino acid tyramine or any supplement that is targeted to increase nitric oxide.*

Feeding the Fire!

The medical profession offers an array of drug treatments for chronic migraine sufferers. For many, unfortunately, the medications prove inadequate to the task. A preventative lifestyle program that focuses on the avoidance of dietary triggers has had the best track record of results. Before eliminating any particular food, it is a good idea to keep a diary to identify specific food triggers and consult with a registered dietitian. Not every known food trigger necessarily brings about a migraine for every migraine sufferer, and therefore a diet should be tailored to the individual. A study of 577 migraine sufferers found cheese, chocolate, red wine, and beer to be the most reported food triggers. With that in mind, here is a list of the most common food triggers to be aware of:

Chocolate. This is a real bummer! The naturally occurring substances in chocolate thought to be responsible for triggering migraines include phenylethylamine, theobromine, and catechin.

Wine and beer and other alcoholic beverages. Tyramine, histamine, phenolics, flavonoids, and sulfites are general triggers of headaches in sensitive individuals. Red wine has more histamine and phenolics than white wine.

Cheese. Aged versions are high in the amino acid tyramine and should be avoided.

Bananas, avocados, broad beans, yogurt, sour cream, and nuts contain tyramine to a lesser degree, but aren't surefire triggers for everyone.

Caffeine is used to constrict blood vessels that are dilated and inflamed. However, many people experience caffeine withdrawal symptoms, such as headaches, when they try to wean themselves off coffee and other caffeinated beverages.

Aspartame. Three double-blind studies have shown a relationship between onset of migraines and frequent versus occasional use of this sweetener.

Nitrites. These are often found in processed meats. Nitric oxide is a vasodilator, which expands the blood vessels—not a good thing for migraines.

MSG. There is some scant research to suggest that high intakes of MSG may bring on migraines.

Fatty foods. Fats in the blood rise during a migraine attack, which can raise inflammatory prostaglandins and cause platelets to stick together and release serotonin, the perfect-storm environment to bring on an attack. A low-fat diet (less than twenty grams a day) has been associated with a significant decrease in headache frequency, intensity, and duration.

Peanuts, yeast, sauerkraut, and aged foods may act as triggers.

MIGRAINE-AVOIDANCE MENU PLAN

Day 1

Breakfast (445)
1 serving *Creamy Cherry Oatmeal* (210) (page 350)
1 cup skim milk (90)
1 kiwi (60)
½ cup orange juice (60)
1 teaspoon honey (25)
1 cup green tea

Lunch (450)
1 serving *Grilled Chicken Salad with Pomegranate Vinaigrette
and Mango Gelée Garnish* (300) (page 324)
1 slice whole wheat sourdough bread (100)
1 cup strawberries (50)
1½ cups water with lemon

Midday Snack (280)
1 serving *Tropical Fruit and Shrimp Gazpacho* (80)
(page 279)
1 serving *Powerhouse Dried Plum Bars* (200) (page 343)
1½ cups sparkling water with lime

Dinner (600)
1 serving *Mango-Tango Tilapia Salad* (270) (page 288)
1 cup steamed Brussels sprouts (60)
½ cup corn polenta (140)
1 serving *Strawberry-Papaya Smoothie* (130) (page 255)

Evening Snack (105)
1 serving *Winter Squash Soup with Roasted Seeds* (70)
(page 277)
1 serving *Watermelon Soda* (36) (page 253)

Day 2

Breakfast (450)
1 serving *Soufflé Omelet with Balsamic Strawberries* (160)
(page 345)
1 serving *Powerhouse Dried Plum Bars* (200) (page 343)
1 cup skim milk (90)

Lunch (400)

1 serving *Curried Chickpeas and Kale* (150) (page 370)

½ cup brown rice (100)

1 serving *Pan-Cooked Apples and Pears in Grape Juice* (150) (page 313)

1½ cups water with lemon

Midday Snack (210)

1 serving *Sharon's Moroccan Couscous* (210) (page 359)

1 cup green tea

Dinner (780)

1 serving *Mediterranean Grilled Mackerel or Bluefish* (250) (page 321)

1 serving *Slow-Cooker Sweet Potatoes* (70) (page 368)

1 serving *Grilled Vidalia Onion and Peach Salad* (270) (page 292)

1 whole grain roll (100)

1 cup skim milk (90)

Evening Snack (140)

1 serving *Fruit and Walnut Jam Conserve* (30) (page 302)

6 rice crackers (110)

1 cup decaffeinated green tea

Day 3

Breakfast (510)

1 serving *Nutty Good Millet Muffins* (240) (page 352)

1-egg veggie omelet (150)

½ cup diced papaya (30)

1 cup skim milk (90)

Lunch (440)
1 serving *Tropical Fruit and Shrimp Gazpacho* (80) (page 279)
1 serving *Raw Kale Salad with Lemon-Honey Vinaigrette* (260)
(page 296)
1 whole grain roll (100)
1½ cups water with lemon

Midday Snack (383)
1 serving *Cherry Zinger Smoothie* (383) (page 256)

Dinner (550)
1 serving *Grilled Chicken Salad with Pomegranate Vinaigrette
and Mango Gelée Garnish* (300) (page 324)
1 serving *Fingerling Potatoes with Asparagus* (250) (page 363)
1½ cups sparkling water with lime

Evening Snack (216)
1 serving *Crumb-Topped Georgia Pecan and Cherry Cereal
Bars* (216) (page 341)
1 cup decaffeinated green tea

Dave's Tips

1. Avoid strong-smelling odors. Colognes, cleaning products, body
   odor, and foul breath can be triggers for migraine sufferers, who
   often have olfactory hypersensitivity (an aversion to strong
   smells).
2. Don't go hungry; eat every three to four hours and drink lots of
   water between meals.
3. Seek out alternative therapies. A review of 150 studies concluded that biofeedback was a very effective tool for managing
   migraine and tension headaches.

MUSCLE PAIN

What Are You Trying to Pull?

Did you know... *strains and sprains account for more than 4.5 million doctor visits every year?*

Optimal Food/Nutrient Highlights

Tart cherries, rose hip tea, caffeine, vitamins C, D, and B complex, selenium, iron.

What Is Muscle Pain?

Muscle aches and pains are common and can involve more than one muscle, ligament, and tendon. Muscle pain can also be a sign of infection (including the flu) or a disorder that affects connective tissues throughout the body (such as lupus).

What Causes It?

Most muscle pain is related to tension, overuse, or muscle injury from exercise. The pain tends to involve specific muscles and starts during or just after the activity. There are many other causes associated with muscle pain, including

Injury or trauma, including sprains and strains.

Drug side effects, such as those from ACE inhibitors for lowering blood pressure and statins for lowering cholesterol.

Electrolyte imbalances, such as having too little potassium or calcium in the diet.

Rheumatologic disorders, such as fibromyalgia, a condition that includes tenderness in the muscles and surrounding soft tissue, sleep difficulties, fatigue, and headaches.

Influenza.

Underlying disease, such as lupus and muscular dystrophy.

How Is Muscle Pain Treated?

As the old saying goes, "An ounce of prevention is worth a pound of cure." When it comes to physical activity, there are a few basic guidelines that reduce risk of muscle injury. You should always warm up and stretch before exercise and maintain adequate hydration during physical activity. Even sitting in the same position most of the day (at a computer, for example) can lead to muscle injury. Try to get up and move and stretch for a little bit at least every hour.

Optimal Life Foods

Tart cherries. College students who drank twelve ounces of a cherry-juice blend twice a day for eight consecutive days had significantly reduced muscle pain after exercise.

Caffeine. In one study, caffeine had a significant effect on reducing leg-muscle-pain ratings after high-intensity exercise in female athletes.

Rose hip tea is a rich source of vitamin C, especially in the powdered form. Flavonoids found in rose hips, such as anthocyanins, have natural anti-inflammatory properties. This herbal tea, made from the fruit of the rose flower (not the rose petals or leaves), helps reduce lower-back pain.

Vitamin B–complex foods. Whole grains, wheat germ, legumes, meat, nuts, oily fish, eggs, dairy, yeast, and most vegetables are great sources for all eight B vitamins.

Selenium-rich foods. Muscle pain, fatigue, and weakness have been reported in patients with selenium deficiency. Foods high in selenium include Brazil nuts, peanuts, fish, wheat, oysters, chicken, and turkey.

Vitamin D– and iron-rich foods. Chronic muscle pain may not improve until underlying depleted tissue-iron stores and vitamin D deficiencies are corrected. Vitamin D food sources include fatty fish, mushrooms, fortified dairy, soy, and orange juice. The better-absorbed heme iron–rich foods include animal proteins such as red meat, especially liver. Other sources of iron include blackstrap molasses, dried plums, figs, and raisins.

Optimal Life Supplements

Vitamin C. In a study of vitamin C supplementation before and after exercise, the subjects who took this vitamin before exercise had reduced muscle soreness after completing their workouts.

Branched-chain amino acids. These are the highest-quality protein building blocks that stimulate muscle repair and growth. Supplementation with branched-chain amino acids prior to squat exercises in test subjects decreased muscle soreness and muscle fatigue that normally occurs for a few days after exercise.

Antioxidant therapy. Supplementation was helpful in one study in reducing muscle soreness in exercisers.

Protease. This is a protein-digestive enzyme that has been shown to reduce soft tissue injury and soreness resulting from intense exercise.

B vitamins. Clinical trials have shown that by supplementing your diet with vitamin B_1, B_6, and B_{12} daily, you can reduce anti-inflammatory medication and lower the chances of further muscle or back pain.

Magnesium. Supplementation with this mineral appears to be of great benefit in relieving muscle tension.

Willow bark. The bark of the white willow tree has pain-relieving properties similar to those of aspirin.

Caution! *Herbal diuretics, such as uva ursi, dandelion root, and red clover tea, are used for mild bloating and fluid retention but are often abused, especially among dieters and athletes. Overuse can deplete fluids and electrolytes in the muscles, resulting in cramping and injury.*

Chinese red rice yeast is a popular dietary supplement for lowering cholesterol. Unfortunately, like statin drugs, one of the side effects of red rice yeast is muscle pain in some individuals.

Feeding the Fire!

Corn, wheat, dairy, citrus, soy, and nuts. Fibromyalgia sufferers have reported a reduction in pain when they've eliminated these allergens from their diets.

Alcohol. Excessive alcohol consumption damages skeletal muscle and can give rise to alcoholic muscle wasting.

MUSCLE-PAIN-RELIEF MENU PLAN

Day 1

Breakfast (395)
1 cup flaxseed cereal flakes (190)
1 cup skim milk (90)
1 cup tart cherries (90)
1 teaspoon honey (25)
1 cup rose hip tea

Lunch (633)
1 serving *Roasted Vegetable and Sweet Swiss Panini* (250)
(page 333)
1 serving *Cherry Zinger Smoothie* (383) (page 256)

Midday Snack (460)
1 serving *Sardine Salad / Dip* (320) (page 265)
12 fat-free corn chips (120)
1½ cups sparkling water with lime

Dinner (500)
4 ounces rotisserie chicken (220)
1 cup steamed Brussels sprouts (60)
1 whole grain roll (100)
2 cups spinach salad with assorted veggies and citrus dressing
(120)
1 cup decaffeinated coffee or tea

Evening Snack (75)
½ cup carrot sticks (25)

2 tablespoons hummus (50)

1 cup decaffeinated green tea

Day 2

Breakfast (466)

1 serving *Crumb-Topped Georgia Pecan and Cherry Cereal
Bars* (216) (page 341)

1 ounce walnuts (160)

1 cup skim milk (90)

Lunch (440)

1 serving *Blackberry Smoothie* (320) (page 258)

1 serving *Avocado-Fennel Citrus Salad* (120) (page 285)

Midday Snack (290)

1 serving *Rosemary Nuts* (290) (page 269)

1 cup green tea

Dinner (474)

1 serving *Cocoa-Encrusted Salmon with Blueberries* (270)
(page 330)

1 serving *Roasted Autumn Vegetables in Sherry Sauce* (114)
(page 360)

1 cup skim milk (90)

Evening Snack (390)

1 serving *Summer Fruits Pie* (390) (page 315)

1 cup decaffeinated green tea

Day 3

Breakfast (488)
1 serving *Triple-Grain Georgia Pecan Pancakes* (188) (page 346)
½ cup hash browns (120)
1 cup tart cherries (90)
1 cup skim milk (90)

Lunch (493)
1 serving *Healthy Turkey Salad Pocket* (233) (page 335)
1 serving *Sharon's Moroccan Couscous* (210) (page 359)
1 cup strawberries (50)
1½ cups water with lemon

Midday Snack (130)
1 serving *Strawberry-Papaya Smoothie* (130) (page 255)

Dinner (646)
1 serving *Chicken Thighs with Red Wine, Dried Plums, and Garlic* (310) (page 323)
1 serving *Sicilian Broccoli Salad* (200) (page 291)
1 whole grain roll (100)
1 serving *Watermelon Soda* (36) (page 253)

Evening Snack (130)
1 serving *Spicy Biscotti* (130) (page 311)
1 serving *Apple-Soy Chai Latte* (130) (page 254)
1 cup rose hip tea

Dave's Tips

1. *Take up yoga.* A study of people with chronic mild lower back pain found there was a significant reduction in pain intensity,

disability, and reliance on pain medication in those who partici-
pated in a yoga class.

2. *Just breathe!* Breathing techniques that make use of the mind-
   body connection have been found to reduce pain. These techniques integrate body awareness, breathing, movement, and
   meditation. One study compared breath therapy with physical
   therapy and found that patients had greater improvements in
   pain management with breath therapy.

3. *Warm up before you work out!* A warm-up performed immediately
   prior to exercise reduces muscle soreness, but cooling down after
   exercise has not been shown to affect muscle soreness either way.

NERVE PAIN

Five Alive

Did you know... *Congress declared in 2001 the beginning of the
"Decade of Pain Control and Research"? They also added pain as
the "fifth vital sign," to accompany blood pressure, temperature,
breathing, and pulse.*

Optimal Food/Nutrient Highlights

Ginger, turmeric, leafy greens, soy, vitamin D, glutamine.

What Is Nerve Pain?

There are three major classifications of nerve pain: neuritis, neuralgia, and neuropathy.

Neuritis is an inflammatory condition of the nerve that results in pain and sensory disturbance. Optic neuritis is inflammation of the optic nerve bundle, which can result in pain and vision loss (temporary or permanent).

Neuralgia is shooting or sudden and recurring pain involving a nerve or group of nerves. It is most common in the elderly but can occur at any age. Trigeminal neuralgia (occurring in the face) is the most common form of neuralgia.

Neuropathy is damage caused to the nerve resulting in burning or shooting pain often accompanied by muscle weakness, numbness, and tingling sensations.

HOW TO TELL IF IT'S NERVE PAIN OR MUSCLE PAIN

You may be suffering from nerve pain if

- The location of the pain doesn't seem to be the result of an event or a physical trauma.
- You experience constant or recurring pain that doesn't seem to go away.
- You feel burning or stabbing pain, you are on pins and needles, and even wearing clothing is painful.
- You're feeling depressed or helpless because normal pain medicine like aspirin does not help stop the pain.

You may be suffering from muscle pain if

- The pain was caused by a physical injury, such as a fall.
- The pain stops once an injury heals.

- Your muscles feel sore and achy.
- You're distressed but hopeful because more pain medicine relieves the pain.*

What Causes It?

There may be several underlying causes, making management of nerve pain difficult.

Neuritis. Optic neuritis often develops as a result of damage caused by a viral-infection-triggered autoimmune response. This is often seen in multiple sclerosis.

Neuralgia. In many cases, the cause is unknown, but neuralgia has been associated with chemical irritation, inflammation, trauma (including surgery), compression of nerves by tumors, and viral infections such as shingles.

Neuropathy. This condition may develop as a side consequence of diseases like cancer (or its treatment) and diabetes or from injury.

Optimal Life Foods

Plenty of whole grains and green leafy vegetables that are rich in B-complex vitamins are essential for nerve health. Other foods rich in B vitamins are wheat germ, figs, nutritional yeast, fruits, and vegetables. Beans are a particularly rich source of B vitamins. Lean meats are an excellent source of vitamin B_{12}. Moderate amounts of mono- and polyunsaturated fats from fish, nuts, and vegetable oils are important for neurological function.

*Adapted from the American Chronic Pain Association website, www.theacpa.org.

Ginger and turmeric. These spices are great anti-inflammatories.

Soy. Foods derived from the soybean have been found to reduce neurological pain in rats, but research has not supported benefits for combating pain in humans thus far.

Optimal Life Supplements

Vitamin D. Supplementation may be an effective "analgesic" in relieving neuropathic pain. And because it is quite difficult to meet your needs with a "safe" level of sun exposure and given that there is a limited array of food choices that are rich in vitamin D, it is a good idea to consider supplementation.

Glutamine. A handful of clinical studies have suggested that oral L-glutamine, an amino acid, may be helpful in reducing symptoms of chemotherapy-induced neuropathy.

Bromelain, boswellia, aswagandha, and turmeric. These are traditional Indian Ayurvedic botanical medicines with strong anti-inflammatory activity. Bromelain is an enzyme derived from pineapple. Boswellia comes from a tree resin similar to frankincense. Aswagandha is a bush whose berries and root are used in Ayurvedic medicine. Turmeric is the yellow spice in curry powder and yellow mustard.

Evening primrose oil. The oil extracted from this wildflower's seeds has been found to be helpful in improving symptoms of neuropathy. In one study, symptoms of numbness, tingling, and loss of sensation in participants with mild diabetic neuropathy were less marked in those who took evening primrose oil than in those who took a placebo.

B_{12}. This important vitamin should be supplemented in the form of sublingual tablets (ones that dissolve under the tongue), because oral supplements are poorly absorbed.

Alpha-lipoic acid. This antioxidant helps the body to produce energy and may decrease the pain of neuritis.

Acetyl-L-carnitine. This vitamin-like antioxidant appears to decrease pain and improve nerve function in people with a nervous-system disorder associated with diabetes (diabetic neuropathy).

Caution! *Dietary supplements containing caffeine or another known herbal stimulant such as guarana may aggravate nerve pain.*

Feeding the Fire!

Caffeine. This stimulant may increase the pain of neuralgia by stimulating the firing of the sensitive trigeminal nerve. Caffeine can prolong the duration of a neuron's activity.

Alcohol can cause further nerve irritation and damage, especially in diabetic neuropathy.

Diets high in saturated and trans fats. These fats can create an environment of inflammation in the body.

NERVE-PAIN-RELIEF MENU PLAN

Day 1

Breakfast (415)
1 serving *Cherry–Chai Spice Granola* (240) (page 348)
1 cup skim milk (90)
½ cup orange juice (60)
1 teaspoon honey (25)
1 cup decaffeinated ginger green tea

Lunch (620)

1 serving *Wild Mushroom Ris-oat-to* (290) (page 357)

1 serving *Curried Chicken-Banana-Yam Soup* (280) (page 280)

1 cup strawberries (50)

Midday Snack (160)

1 serving *Barley Salad with Edamame* (160) (page 287)

Dinner (640)

4 ounces rotisserie chicken (220)

1 serving *Garlic Pipérade Soup* (150) (page 274)

2 cups spinach salad with assorted veggies and citrus dressing (120)

1 serving *Pan-Cooked Apples and Pears in Grape Juice* (150) (page 313)

1½ cups water with lemon

Evening Snack (180)

1 serving *"Devils on Horseback"* (180) (page 270)

1 cup decaffeinated green tea

Day 2

Breakfast (466)

1 serving *Crumb-Topped Georgia Pecan and Cherry Cereal Bars* (216) (page 341)

1 ounce mixed nuts (160)

1 cup skim milk (90)

Lunch (440)

1 serving *Blackberry Smoothie* (320) (page 258)

1 serving *Avocado-Fennel Citrus Salad* (120) (page 285)

Midday Snack (220)
1 serving *Potato-Corn Chowder* (220) (page 273)
1 cup decaffeinated green tea

Dinner (790)
1 serving *Irish Poached Salmon* (350) (page 320)
1 serving *Fingerling Potatoes with Asparagus* (250)
(page 363)
1 whole grain roll (100)
1 cup skim milk (90)

Evening Snack (110)
1 serving *Beanie-Greenie Brownies* (110) (page 309)
1 cup decaffeinated green tea

Day 3

Breakfast (470)
1 serving *Soufflé Omelet with Balsamic Strawberries* (160)
(page 345)
1 turkey sausage link (140)
1 slice whole wheat toast (80)
1 cup skim milk (90)

Lunch (620)
1 serving *Christine's Yummy Bean and Cheese Tostada* (260)
(page 319)
1 serving *Raw Kale Salad with Lemon-Honey Vinaigrette* (260)
(page 296)
1 whole grain roll (100)
1½ cups water with lemon

Midday Snack (230)
1 serving *Quick Pumpkin Smoothie* (230) (page 256)

Dinner (536)
1 serving *Grilled Chicken Salad with Pomegranate Vinaigrette and Mango Gelée Garnish* (300) (page 324)
1 serving *Asparagus-Sesame Stir-Fry* (100) (page 362)
1 whole grain roll (100)
1 serving *Watermelon Soda* (36) (page 253)

Evening Snack (190)
1 serving *Zucchini-Cranberry Muffins* (190) (page 339)
1 cup decaffeinated green tea

Dave's Tips

Try acupuncture. There is good evidence in support of the use of acupuncture and acupressure for pain.

PART 4

IT'S ALL ABOUT PERFORMANCE

MENTAL PERFORMANCE

COGNITIVE DECLINE

Forget About It!

Did you know... *according to the Alzheimer's Association, someone develops Alzheimer's disease every seventy seconds?*

Optimal Food/Nutrient Highlights

Tea, wine, chocolate, grapes, strawberries, blueberries, coffee, fatty fish, turmeric, chewing gum, phosphatidylserine.

What Is Cognitive Decline?

Cognitive decline refers to memory loss and is a normal part of the aging process. But how fast it progresses may depend on a variety of factors. Several aspects of cognitive decline are within our control; others are beyond our influence.

Mild cognitive impairment is often the first stage during which some memory loss, slowing down, and occasional confusion may become evident to the individual and her family and friends. Memory loss is the most common sign of cognitive impairment, but other thought processes can be affected, including communication skills (speech and writing), judgment and decision making, and attention span.

Dementia. Rather than one single disease, *dementia* describes a group of illnesses that involve a loss of brain function. Dementia is a progressive condition that affects about 3.4 million Americans aged seventy-one years and older; somewhere in the neighborhood of 2.4 million of these older Americans are specifically diagnosed with Alzheimer's disease. Signs of dementia are often characterized by these symptoms:

- Confusion, disorientation, or an inability to concentrate
- A slow loss of memory, judgment, or intellectual function
- Personality changes or lack of spontaneity
- Decrease of movement, sensation, speech, hearing, vision, or other brain functions
- Language difficulties

- Loss of bladder control
- Hallucinations and delusions
- Impaired recognition (agnosia)
- Altered sleep patterns

What Causes Dementia?

Dementia is associated with damage to the brain or structural changes within the brain. The list of potential causes is quite long. You can find a wealth of information at the websites of the National Institutes of Health and the National Institute on Aging (both addresses are provided in the resources section at the back of the book).

Optimal Life Foods

Black and green tea. Compounds such as flavonoids, theanine, and caffeine, found in both black and green tea, have been associated with decreased risk of dementia and Alzheimer's disease.

Wine. Too much alcohol consumption increases risk of dementia, yet plant chemicals known as polyphenols, particularly resveratrol found in red wine, may help fight dementia and Alzheimer's disease. The important caveat is to consume wine in moderation.

Chocolate. Research on cocoa flavanols points to increased blood flow to the brain and improved cognition. Surprisingly, a higher cocoa content does not always guarantee the presence of cocoa flavanols. Look for products that boast of their cocoa flavanol content.

Put them all together. A study of elderly Norwegians found that those who consumed chocolate, wine, and tea had better cognitive performance compared with those who didn't partake in any or consumed only one or two of the three.

Concord grape juice. Results from a placebo-controlled human study showed that participants who drank Concord grape juice experienced significant improvement in short-term retention and spatial memory testing.

Blueberries. An animal research study showed significant cognitive improvement in adult mice who consumed wild blueberry (lowbush) concentrate.

Coffee. A Finnish study of over 1,400 subjects found that those who were coffee drinkers at midlife were less likely to develop dementia than those who didn't drink coffee. Those at lowest risk were three-to-five-cup-a-day coffee drinkers!

Omega-3 fatty acids. In a study of 3,660 people over the age of sixty-five, one group ate fish rich in omega-3 fats three times a week or more. A second group didn't eat fish regularly. The fish-eating subjects had over a 25 percent reduction in the risk of silent infarcts of the brain that are associated with dementia.

Strawberries. Researchers at the Jean Mayer USDA Human Nutrition Research Center on Aging at Tufts University demonstrated that strawberry extract helped slow decline in cognitive function.

Turmeric/curry. In a study of over 1,000 elderly Asian subjects, those who reported consuming curry "occasionally to very often" had significantly better Mini-Mental State Examination (MMSE) scores for three categories compared with those subjects who reported they "never or rarely" consumed curry.

Chewing gum. Research conducted by Todd Parish, MD, director of the Center for Advanced Magnetic Resonance Imaging at Northwestern University, found that gum chewing increased blood flow to the brain, decreased emotional stress, and improved cognitive performance.

Optimal Life Supplements

Phosphatidylserine belongs to a group of substances called phospholipids and can be found in the brain as well as in soy and eggs. One study showed improvement in the games of young golfers who took the supplement over a forty-two-day period. Phosphatidylserine is believed to positively affect cognitive function, specifically concentration; however, research does not (yet) support its use for improving cognition in older folks.

B-complex vitamins, including vitamins B_{12}, niacin, and thiamine, are known to improve cognitive performance.

Ginkgo biloba. Researchers at the University of California, Los Angeles, had good results with studies on ginkgo for memory boosting.

Ginseng. Several clinical studies have reported that Panax (Asian) ginseng can improve thinking or learning.

Feeding the Fire!

Alcohol in excess over many years (chronic alcoholism).

Excess sodium linked to hypertension is a risk factor for dementia.

A *diet high in saturated and trans fats.*

Excess calories leading to obesity.

Elevated blood glucose. Researchers at Columbia University found that "senior moments" could in part be blamed on rising (poorly controlled) blood glucose as we age. Maintaining blood glucose, even if you are nondiabetic, could help maintain aspects of cognitive health.

COGNITIVE IMPROVEMENT MENU PLAN

Chew gum between meals and snacks!

Day 1

Breakfast (525)
1 serving *Capp-oat-ccino Delight* (340) (page 337)
1 cup skim milk (90)
4 ounces Concord grape juice (70)
1 teaspoon honey (25)
1 cup coffee

Lunch (570)
1 serving *Wild Mushroom Ris-oat-to* (290) (page 357)
1 serving *Curried Chicken-Banana-Yam Soup* (280)
(page 280)
1½ cups iced tea

Midday Snack (192)
½ serving *Cherry Zinger Smoothie* (192) (page 256)

Dinner (560)
4 ounces roasted turkey with 1 serving *Avocado Chimichurri*
sauce (page 300) (320)
½ cup corn polenta (120)
2 cups spinach salad with assorted veggies and citrus dressing
(120)
1½ cups water with lemon

Evening Snack (180)
1 serving *"Devils on Horseback"* (180) (page 270)
1 cup decaffeinated green tea

Day 2

Breakfast (466)
1 serving *Crumb-Topped Georgia Pecan and Cherry Cereal Bars* (216) (page 341)
1 ounce mixed nuts (160)
1 cup skim milk (90)

Lunch (333)
1 serving *Strawberry-Papaya Smoothie* (130) (page 255)
1 serving *Avocado-Fennel Citrus Salad* (120) (page 285)
1 cup blueberries (83)
1 cup green tea

Midday Snack (210)
1 serving *Asparagus-Carrot Rolls* (210) (page 361)
1 cup green tea

Dinner (760)
1 serving *Potato-Corn Chowder* (220) (page 273)
1 serving *Irish Poached Salmon* (350) (page 320)
1 whole grain roll (100)
1 cup skim milk (90)

Evening Snack (240)
1 serving *Nutty Good Millet Muffins* (240) (page 352)
1 cup decaffeinated green tea

Day 3

Breakfast (453)
1 serving *Soufflé Omelet with Balsamic Strawberries* (160)
(page 345)
½ cup hash browns (120)
1 cup blueberries (83)
1 cup skim milk (90)

Lunch (520)
1 serving *Curried Chickpeas and Kale* (150) (page 370)
2 cups spinach salad with 1 serving *Sweet Vidalia Onion Slaw
with Fennel, Cucumber, and Champagne-Orange Dressing*
(page 297) (270)
1 whole grain roll (100)
1½ cups water with lemon

Midday Snack (290)
1 serving *Strawberry-Papaya Smoothie* (130) (page 255)
1 serving *Raspberry-Yogurt Muffins* (160) (page 338)

Dinner (590)
1 serving *Cocoa-Encrusted Salmon with Blueberries* (270)
(page 330)
1 serving *Asparagus-Sesame Stir-Fry* (100) (page 362)
½ cup brown rice (100)
5 ounces red wine (optional) (120)
1 cup decaffeinated green tea

Evening Snack (153)
½ serving *Healthy Turkey Salad Pocket* (117) (page 335)
1 serving *Watermelon Soda* (36) (page 253)

Dave's Tips

1. Maintaining good muscle mass and strength and a healthy body weight helps keep the mind sound. Exercise keeps blood glucose managed better.
2. Keeping sodium down and potassium up by eating more fruits and vegetables helps manage blood pressure.
3. Sudoku, crossword puzzles, and brain teasers help keep your mind flexible.

DEPRESSION

Bummer!

Did you know...*depression affects over 120 million people worldwide of all ages and backgrounds?*

Optimal Food/Nutrient Highlights

Fatty fish, folate, tryptophan, zinc, vitamin D.

What Is Depression?

According to the World Health Organization, "Depression is a common mental disorder that presents with depressed mood, loss of interest or pleasure, feelings of guilt or low self-worth, disturbed sleep or appetite, low energy, and poor concentration. These problems can become chronic or recurrent and lead to substantial impairments in an individual's ability to take care of his or her everyday responsibilities. At its worst, depression can lead to suicide, a tragic fatality associated with the loss of about 850,000 lives every year." It is also one of the leading causes of disability worldwide.

There are various categories of depression.

Major depression. This can include symptoms such as sadness, loss of interest or pleasure in activities that you once enjoyed, change in weight (gain or loss), poor sleep, undersleeping or oversleeping, energy loss, feelings of worthlessness, and thoughts of death or suicide.

Dysthymia. People with dysthymia are described as mildly depressed on most days for at least two years. They experience similar but less severe symptoms of major depression.

Seasonal affective disorder. People affected by SAD deal with many of the symptoms of major depression on a recurrent basis during the wintertime.

Postpartum depression. Women may experience this form of depression within the first few months of giving birth. The symptoms are identical to those of major depression and often interfere with the mother's ability or desire to take care of herself and her newborn.

Bipolar disorder. This illness was previously known in the psychiatric profession as manic depression. Many people continue to refer to individuals who suffer from this debilitating disorder as manic-depressives. In this disorder, feelings of deep depression can be replaced with feelings of extreme elation, sometimes within the same day. People with bipolar disorder are often thought of as being moody.

There is also a category called "treatment resistant" depression, in which, despite all efforts, depressive symptoms continue on.

What Causes Depression?

Depression seems to be multifactorial. The root of depression is an imbalance of brain chemicals called neurotransmitters, specifically the brain chemicals serotonin, dopamine, noradrenaline, and gamma-aminobutyric acid (GABA). However, there may be many underlying factors involved that trigger this imbalance. A helping professional will want to know about

Family history. Depression has been found to run in families for generations.

Trauma and stress. Financial woes, death of a loved one, divorce, retirement, and beginning or losing a job are just a few life-changing events that can trigger depression.

A gloomy outlook. Those who tend to look at the glass as being half empty or adopt a negative outlook on life are at higher risk of depression. (This may also be the classic "Which came first...?" because a negative outlook is also a sign of depression.)

Physical conditions. Serious medical conditions are often accompanied and exacerbated by depression, partly because of the physical weakness and stress they bring on. Depression can further weaken the immune system and increase sensitivity to pain. Sometimes the treatment for severe illness itself, such as side effects of medication, can bring about depression.

Additional psychological disorders. Anxiety, eating disorders, schizophrenia, and substance abuse often appear along with depression.

Depression may be treated with psychotherapy (talk therapy) and antidepressants.

Optimal Life Foods

Omega 3–rich foods. Epidemiological studies have shown a positive association between diets lacking in adequate levels of omega-3 fats and mood disorders such as depression and schizophrenia. Fish, flaxseed, walnuts, pumpkin seeds, and canola oil are good sources.

Folate-rich foods. Impaired levels of folate have been associated with poor cognition and depression. Good food sources of folate include spinach, beans, orange juice, hazelnuts (which contain the highest concentration of folate of all of the tree nuts), avocados, and wheat germ.

Tryptophan-rich foods. Tryptophan is an amino acid that helps produce the feel-good and sleep-better neurotransmitter serotonin. Good sources include chicken, turkey, beef, lamb, dairy (milk, yogurt, cheese, eggs), soy, spelt, nuts, beans, tuna, and salmon.

Foods rich in zinc. Animal research has shown depressive behavior associated with poor zinc intake in the diet. Stock up on oysters, beef, chicken, Cheddar cheese, yogurt, beans, Brazil nuts, basil, pumpkin seeds, and whole and fortified grains.

Vitamin D–rich foods may also have an anti-inflammatory effect and increase the flexibility of cell membranes, which makes the brain's neurotransmitters work better. While primarily generated after the skin soaks up the sun's UVB rays, vitamin D can be obtained from oily fish, mushrooms, and supplemented products like cow's milk or soy milk and orange juice.

Optimal Life Supplements

Fish oil. A randomized, controlled study showed significant improvement in measures of depression for middle-aged women who were taking an omega-3 supplement compared with a placebo.

Vitamin D. A double-blind study showed marked improvement in depressed individuals with low blood levels of vitamin D who took high-dose vitamin D supplements compared with a placebo. However, another study showed that brain lesions were associated with high vitamin D and calcium intake. Bottom line—seek the guidance of a registered dietitian or a physician if you are going to take more than the daily recommendation for vitamin D.

5-hydroxytryptophan. This amino acid may help restore serotonin in the brain. There is a small body of research that has demonstrated reduced feelings of panic and depression with this supplement. But beware that 5-HTP may interfere with other antidepressants or medications. Consult with your doctor before adding 5-HTP to your regimen.

Saint-John's-wort. This herb has been touted for helping with mild depression. Many studies support that it may be as effective as some commonly prescribed antidepressants for mild depression. However, two major studies by the National Center for Complementary and Alternative Medicine demonstrated that Saint-John's-wort was no more effective than a placebo in treating more severe forms of depression.

CoQ_{10}. Both cholesterol-lowering statin drugs and tricyclic antidepressants lower coenzyme Q_{10}. This is a double whammy if my patients are on both, which they often are. Supplementation of CoQ_{10} may be necessary if you are on these medications.

Caution! *Many supplements and drugs, including Saint-John's-wort, diet pills, SAMe, and 5-HTP, may interfere with antidepressants. Consult with a registered dietitian or your pharmacist to find out more on food-supplement and medication interactions.*

Feeding the Fire!

Trans and saturated fats. These fats do not feed your brain what it needs. In fact, they have been implicated in making the membranes within the brain so rigid that they prevent brain chemicals called neurotransmitters from getting in where they are needed most.

Poor glycemic control. A lab measure of whether your body is doing a good job of managing blood glucose is called hemoglobin A1C. Studies show that diabetics who have higher levels of glucose also have higher rates of depression than those who have better glycemic control.

Low-carb, high-protein diets? In one study, female cyclists became more depressed on a low-carb diet than on a medium- or high-carb diet. Other research is mixed on this subject. My observation is that anyone who feels like they are going to be saddled with a deprivation diet (of any kind) for the rest of their life will wind up not being a happy camper. Your brain needs glucose to make serotonin, so dipping too low in your carb intake may be a formula for unhappiness. The menu plan on page 85 has plenty of the kind of carbs that are best for your physical and mental health.

Alcohol. Although it may make you feel happier initially, alcohol is a depressant drug that dulls the senses and reduces serotonin levels in the brain.

Avoid tyramine-containing foods if you are taking monoamine oxidase inhibitors (MAOIs). MAOIs are a category of antidepressants that help keep neurotransmitter levels high in the brain. But tyramine, an amino acid naturally found in the diet, can react negatively with MAOIs and should be avoided, because it may cause a sharp increase in blood pressure, which could lead to stroke. Some tyramine-rich foods to avoid include aged cheeses, beer, wine, pickles, and broad beans. For a more comprehensive list, ask a registered dietitian, your pharmacist, or your doctor.

Skipping meals. Your goal is to keep blood glucose steady. Erratic eating may trigger anxiety, panic, anger, and depressed feelings.

GET HAPPY MENU PLAN

Those of you who are on monoamine oxidase inhibitor medications may notice that I have not provided a tyramine-restricted diet. Drug-nutrient interaction is an important consideration. While aged cheeses, beer, wine, pickles, and broad beans (to name a few of the tyramine-rich foods) are not prevalent in this menu plan, it is certainly not tyramine-free. Work with a registered dietitian or pharmacist to tweak these meals if you are taking MAOI medications.

Day 1

Breakfast (425)
1 serving *Capp-oat-ccino Delight* (340) (page 337)
½ cup orange juice (vitamin D fortified) (60)
1 teaspoon honey (25)
1 cup green tea

Lunch (410)
2 servings *Kale Balls* (80) (page 262)
1 serving *Curried Chicken-Banana-Yam Soup* (280)
(page 280)
1 cup strawberries (50)
1½ cups water with lemon

Midday Snack (230)
1 serving *Quick Pumpkin Smoothie* (230) (page 256)

Dinner (697)
4 ounces roasted turkey with 1 serving *Avocado Chimichurri* sauce (page 300) (320)
1 serving *Winter White Bean Chili* (257) (page 282)
2 cups spinach salad with assorted veggies and citrus dressing (120)
1½ cups water with lemon

Evening Snack (240)
1 serving *Nutty Good Millet Muffins* (240) (page 352)
1 cup decaffeinated green tea

Day 2

Breakfast (460)
1 serving *Chef Wiley's Granola* (290) (page 351)
1 cup light soy milk (110)
½ cup orange juice (vitamin D fortified) (60)

Lunch (463)
1 serving *Healthy Turkey Salad Pocket* (233) (page 335)
1 serving *Japanese-Style Vegetable Fried Rice* (230) (page 355)
1 cup green tea

Midday Snack (330)
½ serving *Sardine Salad / Dip* (160) (page 265)
1 whole wheat pita cut into triangles (170)
1½ cups water with lemon

Dinner (540)
1 serving *Dilled Salmon Cakes* (180) (page 328)
2 cups spinach salad with 1 serving *Sweet Vidalia Onion Slaw
with Fennel, Cucumber, and Champagne-Orange Dressing*
(page 297) (270)
1 cup skim milk (90)

Evening Snack (180)
1 ounce hazelnuts (180)
1 cup decaffeinated green tea

Day 3

Breakfast (390)
1 serving *Soufflé Omelet with Balsamic Strawberries* (160)
(page 345)
1 slice whole wheat toast (80)
½ cup orange juice (vitamin D fortified) (60)
1 cup skim milk (90)

Lunch (500)
1 serving *Curried Chickpeas and Kale* (150) (page 370)
1 serving *Nuts and Berry Fruit Salad* (350) (page 286)
1½ cups water with lemon

Midday Snack (192)
½ serving *Cherry Zinger Smoothie* (192) (page 256)

Dinner (740)
1 serving *Gazpacho* (130) (page 275)

1 serving *Cocoa-Encrusted Salmon with Blueberries* (270)
(page 330)
1 serving *Sharon's Moroccan Couscous* (210) (page 359)
1 serving *Apple-Soy Chai Latte* (130) (page 254)

Evening Snack (176)
2 servings *Cheese-and-Fruit Kebabs* (140) (page 272)
1 serving *Watermelon Soda* (36) (page 253)

Elizabeth Somer's Tips for Boosting Mood
Elizabeth Somer, MA, RD, is a registered dietitian and an award-winning writer, having authored nine books, most notably Food and Mood.

1. Eat breakfast. I am frequently asked what a person should eat midday to boost mood. But if that person has skipped breakfast, there is nothing that can make up for not eating that meal. Start the day off right with whole grains, a small amount of protein, and a good amount of fruit. An example would be a bowl of whole grain cereal, soy milk, and a large bowl of fruit.
2. Avoid or limit quick fixes such as caffeine, refined grains, and refined sugar.
3. Drink lots of water.
4. Eat a light lunch and dinner and have a small all-carbohydrate snack before bedtime, such as air-popped popcorn or half of an English muffin and fruit jam, to boost serotonin levels so you can sleep soundly.
5. Take a multivitamin to fill the gaps on the days you don't eat perfectly.
6. My other favorite supplement includes fish oil or a docosahexaenoic acid (DHA) supplement that supplies at least 200 mg of DHA.

7. Exercise! Exercise! Exercise! People who engage in vigorous activity daily are the least likely to be depressed.

8. Surround yourself with happy people—the mood rubs off! Monitor your self-talk so you don't repeat negative, defeating mantras. Lastly, be eternally grateful for all you have and have been given.

STRESS AND ANXIETY

eGAD!

Did you know... *generalized anxiety disorder (GAD) affects nearly 7 million adult Americans, and that nearly twice as many women suffer from this illness as men?*

Optimal Food/Nutrient Highlights

Tea, chamomile, celery, cilantro, oranges, chicken, sunflower seeds, mushrooms, theanine, B-complex vitamins.

What Are Stress and Anxiety?

Stress. Every human on earth has experienced some degree of stress at one time or another in their lives. The amazing thing about stress is that not all health experts agree on it as being a *bad* thing. On the positive side, the daily stress we encounter can get us out of dangerous situations, by alerting us not to do battle with an oncoming truck we just noticed, and also by motivating us to achieve greater things by taking risks. Ultimately, we can reap tremendous rewards having gone through stressful experiences like writing a book, winning an election, passing an exam—all can be well worth the perceived *ordeal*. However, when stress becomes unmanageable, unbearable, and takes over our lives, it is no longer an asset but instead negatively affects our physical and mental well-being. And that may be the one thing that the experts can agree on: Feeling out of control is *not* a good thing.

Unmanaged stress often takes the form of profound fatigue, insomnia, anger, irritability, and constant mind-chatter—that constant *worrying* that gets in the way of living. Unmanaged stress has also been linked to severe medical problems such as high blood pressure, pain, irritable bowel syndrome and other digestive disorders, immune impairment, and even the speeding up of the aging process of the brain.

Generalized anxiety disorder (GAD) is a more extreme stress disorder characterized by constant fear, anxiety, worry, and a feeling of being tense, whether having a good reason to justify that feeling or not. Some physical manifestations of this condition include sleep disturbances, shakiness and trembling, muscle aches and pain, profuse sweating, cold and clammy hands, feeling dizzy, feeling tired, rapid heart rate or feeling that your heart is pounding out of your chest, dry mouth, upset stomach, diarrhea, and shortness of breath.

Post-traumatic stress disorder (PTSD) is another debilitating illness that can result from having gone through a traumatic event such as a war, being a victim of a crime, or having survived a natural or unnatural disaster (such as 9/11). It was originally observed in war vets experiencing battle fatigue that was once referred to as shell shock. Those who have PTSD often "relive" their experience in the form of nightmares or even waking flashbacks.

Daily-life scenarios can trigger flashbacks. Being in a tight space such as an elevator or feeling confined when undergoing an MRI test or finding yourself in a situation where there is a sense of loss of control can trigger the illusion that the traumatic event is happening again.

What Causes Stress and Anxiety?

Just like the daunting task of defining what *stress* actually means to every individual, the process of identifying the causes of stress can be subjective and varied. What causes stress for one person may be a cause of elation for another: Giving a speech, riding on a roller coaster, and climbing to the top of the executive ladder are a few examples that can bring great joy or sheer terror. There may be genetic factors at play, and certainly environmental stressors can make a stress load unbearable. There can be an imbalance in chemicals in the brain that can predispose one to being less capable of handling stress, as well.

Optimal Life Foods

Malnutrition can put an added layer of stress on the body by weakening the immune system and creating inflammatory conditions that make you more vulnerable to disease. Taking in too many calories can translate to an increased physical burden of dragging around too much weight. The brain is an organ also deserving of the right fuel to make it work correctly.

Tea is rich in the amino acid theanine, which has been found to increase GABA and dopamine, both neurotransmitters in the brain that exert a calming effect.

Chamomile tea is an age-old herb for producing calm and relaxation.

Celery. Besides being a great veggie to snack on that provides crunch and is a low-cal alternative for nervous eaters, celery contains flavonoids and antioxidant compounds that help halt oxidative stress in the body.

Cilantro (coriander). Cilantro was long used in Iranian folk medicine for the relief of stress and anxiety; now modern medicine has shown an association with mood. An animal study demonstrated that cilantro had sedative and muscle-relaxant qualities.

Oranges. In addition to their great vitamin C content, helpful in protecting the body against the ravages of stress, just getting a whiff has been shown to reduce anxiety and improve mood in patients waiting in a dentist's office.

Chicken, tuna, salmon, and mushrooms are rich in niacin, otherwise known as vitamin B_3, which is a very important vitamin for energy production. Vitamin B_3 also helps support the neurotransmission system of the brain that diminishes depression and anxiety.

Sunflower seeds, black beans, and yellow corn are rich in thiamin, also known as vitamin B_1. These foods help your body by providing energy and coordinating the activity of nerves and muscles. Low levels of thiamin have been associated with restlessness and irritability.

Bell peppers, spinach, and bananas are great sources of vitamin B_6. This vitamin supports the nervous system and can assist your body in fighting feelings of anxiety and panic.

Meat, fish, and yogurt all contain vitamin B_{12}. This is a vital nutrient that promotes proper development of nerve cells. Heart palpitations and fatigue are often seen in anxiety patients and may be associated with low levels of B_{12}.

Halibut, salmon, sesame seeds, pumpkin seeds, Swiss chard, al-monds, soy, and spinach are all rich in the mineral magnesium. Including these foods in your diet may be instrumental in keeping the effects of both physical and emotional stress at bay.

Optimal Life Supplements

Theanine. This substance found in tea has calming effects and mood-enhancing properties and now can be found in enhanced sport beverages and dietary supplements.

5-hydroxytryptophan. Derived from the seed of the African plant *Griffonia simplifica,* 5-HTP may help relieve panic attacks.

Magnesium aids in overall relaxation.

B-complex vitamins are key in carbohydrate metabolism to produce energy and calm nerves.

Calcium has been found to induce relaxation and reduce irritability.

Caution! *Highly caffeinated supplements and herbal stimulants spur on stress and anxiety.*

Feeding the Fire!

Alcohol acts as a depressive drug in the body. Unfortunately, those who feel stressed often turn to alcohol to help relieve their burdens. This can leave one feeling more depressed and contribute to a vicious cycle, as is true with any other addictive substance.

Both caffeine (in high amounts) and nicotine can also worsen feelings of anxiety.

Skipping meals or eating meals that are mostly comprised of refined carbohydrates may send blood glucose crashing down, which often triggers anxiety, panic attacks, and feelings of stress.

RELAXING MENU PLAN

Day 1

Breakfast (425)
1 cup flaxseed cereal flakes (190)
1 cup skim milk (90)
½ medium banana (60)
4 ounces orange juice (60)
1 teaspoon honey (25)
1 cup decaffeinated green tea

Lunch (515)
1 deli sandwich made with bell pepper slices, spinach, tomatoes, breast of chicken, and Dijon mustard on sesame-rye bread (335)
12 fat-free corn chips (120)
1 kiwi (60)
1 cup chamomile tea

Midday Snack (260)
1 cup low-fat vanilla yogurt layered with ½ cup mixed berries and topped with ½ serving *Cherry–Chai Spice Granola* (page 348) (260)
1½ cups sparkling water with lime

Dinner (670)
4 ounces grilled tuna with 1 serving *Avocado Chimichurri* sauce (page 300) (290)

1 serving *Quinoa Pilaf with Currants and Turmeric* (320)
(page 369)
2 cups spinach salad with cilantro and 1 serving *Creamy Avocado Dressing* (page 306) (60)
1 cup decaffeinated green tea

Evening Snack (180)
½ cup celery sticks (25)
1 tablespoon sunflower butter (95)
1 apple (60)
1 cup decaffeinated green tea

Day 2

Breakfast (440)
2 scrambled (omega-3 enriched) eggs (150)
1 whole grain English muffin (100)
1 cup Concord grapes (100)
1 cup skim milk (90)

Lunch (328)
1 serving *Chile-Honey Almond Chicken Kebabs* (261) (page 266)
2 cups romaine or leaf-lettuce salad with 1 serving *Creamy Avocado Dressing* (page 306) (60)
1 orange (60)
1½ cups decaffeinated iced green tea

Midday Snack (320)
2 ounces trail mix (almonds, pumpkin seeds, sunflower seeds, cranberries) (320)

Dinner (615)
1 serving *Irish Poached Salmon* (350) (page 320)
1 serving *Roasted Root Vegetables* (240) (page 365)
1 teaspoon honey (25)
1 cup decaffeinated green tea

Evening Snack (350)
½ cup avocado guacamole (230)
12 fat-free corn chips (120)
1 cup decaffeinated green tea

Day 3

Breakfast (503)
1 serving *Triple-Grain Georgia Pecan Pancakes* (188)
(page 346) topped with 1 tablespoon sunflower seeds (45)
1 omega-3 egg–veggie omelet with corn, spinach, and red
peppers (100)
1 orange (60)
1 cup light soy milk (110)

Lunch (580)
1 serving *Mango-Tango Tilapia Salad* (270) (page 288)
2 servings *Kale Balls* (80) (page 262)
1 serving *Quick Pumpkin Smoothie* (230) (page 256)
1½ cups iced green tea

Midday Snack (205)
½ almond butter and apricot jam sandwich on whole grain
flaxseed bread (205)
1½ cups water

Dinner (520)
1 serving *Christine's Yummy Bean and Cheese Tostada* (260)
(page 319)
1 serving *Gazpacho* (130) (page 275)
1 serving *Strawberry-Papaya Smoothie* (130) (page 255)

Evening Snack (142)
½ serving *Healthy Turkey Salad Pocket* (117) (page 335)
1 teaspoon honey (25)
1 cup chamomile tea

Dave's Tips

1. Try yoga, meditation, prayer, or deep breathing for ten minutes upon waking and before retiring for the evening.
2. Start a physical activity program to help you relax and burn off stress. Take a class at the YMCA, join a reading group, take up knitting. Interacting socially with people can do wonders for your mood.
3. Identify and avoid situations that create stress and bring on panic attacks.
4. Stop negative thinking. Find out about cognitive-behavorial therapy and other psychological treatments that can help you to break negative rumination and other debilitating thought traps.

INSOMNIA

That's a bunch of CPAP!

Did you know... most adults have experienced insomnia or sleeplessness at one time or another in their lives? It is estimated that 30 to 50 percent of the general population is affected by insomnia regularly. The rise in the use of continuous positive airway pressure (CPAP) machines, an aide to help a condition called sleep apnea often associated with obesity, is up 96 percent since 2004!

Optimal Food/Nutrient Highlights

Walnuts, cherries, dairy, turkey, lettuce, chamomile, B-complex vitamins.

What Is Insomnia?

Insomnia is a health condition that causes difficulties in initiating and/or maintaining sleep. The three categories of insomnia are based on the length of time that you suffer with it:

Transient insomnia generally occurs less than once a week.

Intermittent insomnia occurs on and off.

Chronic insomnia occurs frequently and lasts for a month or more.

Though it is a nighttime problem, its true effects are often manifested in the daytime by causing fatigue, poor concentration, moodiness and depression, and increased accidents.

What Causes It?

Insomnia can be a symptom of underlying physical or emotional challenges that may be transient or chronic in nature. Transient insomnia causes include jet lag, changes in work schedule, feeling too hot or cold in the bedroom, feeling stressed, the burden of illness, and overuse of drugs, including alcohol, sedatives, and stimulants. A common side effect of some medications, even if taken as directed, is insomnia.

Chronic or long-term insomnia has many of the same causes as transient insomnia, especially psychological reasons—most notably anxiety and stress. Sleep is also impacted by chronic pain; chronic fatigue syndrome; heart and pulmonary disease; acid reflux disease (GERD); obstructive sleep apnea; Parkinson's, Alzheimer's, and multiple sclerosis; brain tumors, strokes, and other traumas to the brain. And, not surprisingly, sleeping with someone who snores!

Optimal Life Foods

Omega-3 fats. Hamsters that ate a diet lacking in omega-3 fats showed more frequent sleep disturbances and greater incidence of attention deficit/hyperactivity disorder in one study.

Chamomile tea and decaffeinated herbal tea are great relaxers before bedtime.

B complex–rich foods. Whole grains, brown rice, oats, and dark green leafy vegetables calm the nervous system.

Complex carbohydrates have a mild sleep-enhancing effect because they increase serotonin, a brain neurotransmitter that promotes sleep. Many carbohydrate-rich foods like whole grains and dark green vegetables are also high in B-complex vitamins.

Lettuce has been used to promote sleep.

Tryptophan-rich foods. Chicken, dairy products, nuts, seeds, bananas, soybeans and soy products, tuna, shellfish, and turkey help the body produce serotonin.

Melatonin-rich foods. Walnuts, tart cherries, brown rice, corn, oats, ginger, tomatoes, bananas, and barley are natural sources of the sleep hormone melatonin. Russel J. Reiter, PhD, a nutrition researcher at the University of Texas Health Science Center and one of the world's leading authorities on melatonin, believes that tart cherries could help regulate the body's natural sleep cycle and decrease the time it takes to fall asleep.

Optimal Life Supplements

Melatonin. This hormone is produced while you are sleeping and is secreted by the pineal gland, located in the brain. Not having adequate exposure to sunlight and also self-electing to stay up late can affect melatonin production. Melatonin supplementation may be beneficial in those with circadian rhythm disorders.

Valerian. A popular herbal product that helps induce sleep, valerian was tested in a double-blind, placebo-controlled study. Valerian extract was shown to significantly improve sleep quality compared with those who were taking a placebo.

Caution! *Any medications or supplements that contain caffeine or herbal stimulants can interrupt sleep.*

Feeding the Fire!

Low-carb diets. A study compared the effect on sleep of consuming a low-carbohydrate diet with a mixed diet in humans. The low-carb-diet followers had less rapid-eye-movement (REM) sleep. High-protein meals can inhibit sleep by blocking the synthesis of serotonin, making us feel more alert.

Alcohol and caffeine. Both cause sleep disturbances.

Eating just before bedtime. Blood is pooled toward the stomach for digestion instead of being used for repair during restful sleep. It is okay to have something light before bedtime, but nothing too heavy.

Gassy foods. Avoid foods that are likely to cause gas, heartburn, or indigestion, such as fatty and spicy foods.

SLEEPING TIME MENU PLAN

Day 1

Breakfast (425)
1 cup flaxseed cereal flakes (190)
1 cup skim milk (90)
1 kiwi (60)
½ cup orange juice (60)
1 teaspoon honey (25)
1 cup decaffeinated green tea

Lunch (556)
1 serving *Roasted Vegetable and Sweet Swiss Panini* (250) (page 333)
1 serving *Crumb-Topped Georgia Pecan and Cherry Cereal Bars* (216) (page 341)
1 cup skim milk (90)
1½ cups water with lemon

Midday Snack (220)
1 serving *Chilean Fruit Guacamole* (100) (page 259)
12 fat-free corn chips (120)
1½ cups sparkling water with lime

Dinner (570)
4 ounces rotisserie chicken (220)
1 serving *Polenta Pizza* (180) (page 329)
½ cup edamame (110)
2 cups spinach salad with assorted veggies and citrus dressing (60)
1 cup water

Evening Snack (320)
2 ounces trail mix (walnuts, dried cherries, toasted soybeans, and dried banana) (320)
1 cup chamomile tea

Day 2

Breakfast (420)
1 serving *Soufflé Omelet with Balsamic Strawberries* (160) (page 345)
½ banana (60)
1 slice whole grain toast with 1 teaspoon *Fruit and Walnut Jam Conserve* (110) (page 302)
1 cup skim milk (90)

Lunch (440)
1 serving *Blackberry Smoothie* (320) (page 258)
1 serving *Avocado-Fennel Citrus Salad* (120) (page 285)

Midday Snack (290)
1 serving *Rosemary Nuts* (290) (page 269)
1 cup decaffeinated green tea

Dinner (670)
1 serving *Mediterranean Grilled Mackerel or Bluefish* (250) (page 321)

1 serving *Japanese-Style Vegetable Fried Rice* (230) (page 355)
1 whole grain roll (100)
1 cup skim milk (90)

Evening Snack (140)
1 serving *Christine's Baked Custard* (140) (page 308)
1 cup decaffeinated green tea

Day 3

Breakfast (360)
1 serving *Creamy Cherry Oatmeal* (210) (page 350)
1 pear (60)
1 cup skim milk (90)

Lunch (440)
1 serving *Tropical Fruit and Shrimp Gazpacho* (80)
(page 279)
1 serving *Raw Kale Salad with Lemon-Honey Vinaigrette* (260)
(page 296)
1 whole grain roll (100)
1½ cups water with lemon

Midday Snack (383)
1 serving *Cherry Zinger Smoothie* (383) (page 256)

Dinner (504)
1 serving *Chile-Honey Almond Chicken Kebabs* (261) (page 266)
1 serving *Sicilian Broccoli Salad* (200) (page 291)
1 serving *Vegetable Pavé with Cauliflower Coulis* (60)
(page 366)
1 serving *Watermelon Soda* (36) (page 253)

Evening Snack (250)
1 serving *Raspberry-Yogurt Muffins* (160) (page 338)
1 cup warm skim milk (90)

Dave's Tips

1. Drink some chamomile tea or a glass of warm milk before going to bed. Keep fluids to a minimum if you tend to get up in the middle of the night.
2. Avoid eating, especially large meals, for at least one hour before retiring for the evening.

PHYSICAL PERFORMANCE

FATIGUE

Sick and Tired

Did you know... over 7 million doctor's office visits per year in the United States are made to address fatigue-related conditions? A survey of workers in the United States found that 38 percent of them complained of fatigue, with an annual cost to employers in lost work estimated at nearly $136 billion.

Optimal Food/Nutrient Highlights

Water, apples, tea, garlic, protein, carbs, iron, vitamin C, carnitine.

What Is Fatigue?

Whether you are a busy mother with children, a power exec, a student with a heavy course load, or just simply one of the millions of Americans who complain that they are tired of being tired, everyone experiences fatigue at one time or another. And constant fatigue gets in the way of peak physical performance, no matter what you do!

Mental fatigue occurs when you feel cognitively challenged after performing mentally taxing tasks. Many often exclaim, "I can't think anymore" when they reach the point of mental fatigue. Researchers also found that those who engage in tasks that are mentally fatiguing can tire more quickly when participating in physical activity.

Physical (general) fatigue is defined as a daily lack of energy or unusual or excessive whole-body tiredness, not relieved by sleep. It can be acute, lasting a month or less, or chronic, lasting from one to six months or longer.

What Causes It?

Fatigue is a normal response to prolonged physical and emotional stress. But if it occurs all of the time, it may be a sign of a more serious psychological or physical challenge that should be evaluated. Some of the most common causes of fatigue are

Lifestyle choices. Inactivity, staying up too late and forgoing sleep, or not eating a healthy, well-balanced diet can lead to feelings of exhaustion.

Stress. Some thrive on it, but most people feel drained from being in a constant state of "fight or flight."

Allergies. Mounting an immune response can sap energy. Imagine how many other daily battles may be draining your energy reserves!

Anemia. The most common form is iron-deficiency anemia. Iron helps red blood cells carry oxygen throughout the body. Many women are anemic and don't even know it.

Depression. See "Depression," page 79.

Pain. See "House of Pain," page 47.

Insomnia. Sleep apnea and other sleep disorders diminish oxygen supply. People who sleep fewer than six hours a night or more than nine are more likely to be obese according to a government study, and being obese requires extra energy to be expended.

Thyroid disorders. Either an underactive or overactive thyroid can contribute to fatigue.

Drug and alcohol use. Alcohol is a depressant, and many drugs (prescription or recreational) have side effects of fatigue.

Anorexia and malnutrition. Inadequate calorie and carbohydrate consumption from fad dieting can contribute to fatigue. During prolonged exercise, energy stores (glycogen) in the muscles can become depleted.

Autoimmune disorders. Some autoimmune disorders, such as pernicious and hemolytic anemia and lupus, affect the oxygen-carrying capacity of red blood cells. Inflammatory conditions like rheumatoid arthritis and disorders that attack the thyroid, including Graves' disease, often present with fatigue as a main complaint.

Cancer causes fatigue; its treatments, such as chemotherapy and radiation therapy, can be exhausting regimens.

Endocrine disorders. One of the earliest medical problems identified in marathon runners suffering from fatigue at the end of a race was hypoglycemia (low blood sugar).

Hypertension. High blood pressure can result in feeling tired.

Medication side effects. High-blood-pressure and cardiac medications, allergy medications, cold formulas, antihistamines, antianxiety medications, and, ironically, stimulant drugs may worsen fatigue in the long run.

Chronic fatigue syndrome. CFS is a condition that mimics flu symptoms and lasts for six months or more.

Dehydration. Cognition and physical ability are very dependent on adequate hydration.

Obesity. An estimated 97 million adults in the United States are overweight or obese. Are we tired because we are fat, or are we fat because we are tired? Research has shown that lack of sleep affects our metabolic rate, and obese people often experience fatigue and decreased physical endurance. A recent study found that certain biochemical markers associated with obesity are altered unfavorably when we are tired—namely, fat-promoting cortisol rises and carnitine, needed for energy production and lean-muscle-mass growth, diminishes.

Optimal Life Foods

Hydration. Technically, water isn't a food, but we couldn't live an optimal (or any) life without it. Sixty to 75 percent of the body's composition is made up of water, so it is no wonder that if we are down a quart or two, it could have a profound effect on our energy levels. By the way, most of the water in the body comes from drinking water and other beverages, and not from the food we eat.

Use these three factors as a best guess to your hydration status. If you experience two out of three, you are dehydrated!

Weight. If you have lost weight, particularly after exercise, it is most likely due to fluid losses.

Urine. If your urine is dark, concentrated, and has a strong odor, that could be a sign of dehydration.

Thirst. This not always the most reliable indicator of hydration, because by the time you are thirsty, you could be well into a dehydrated state.

Daily intake of nonfood sources of fluids should be about thirteen cups for males and about nine cups for females (more if pregnant or breast-feeding). Ironically, recent research has noted that the more physically active Americans become, the less fluid they consume. Bottom line: Start drinking!

Carbohydrates. Whole grains, vegetables, fruits, and dairy all supply needed carbohydrates, the fuel your body prefers to run on.

Protein. Foods rich in protein like fish, lean meats, beans, and dairy products help keep blood glucose stable, and not rising and falling like a roller coaster.

Apples. Polyphenols found in apples improved physical performance and combated fatigue in one study.

Garlic. Animal and human studies have shown that garlic promotes endurance during exercise and has an antifatigue effect.

Green tea. Epigallocatechin-3-gallate (EGCG) is a significant antioxidant that occurs naturally in green tea. An animal study found rats who were stressed and fed an extract of EGCG had marked improvement in both physical and mental energy.

Iron-rich foods. Clams, liver, oysters, beef, shrimp, sardines, turkey, enriched cereals, beans, pumpkin seeds, potatoes with skins, asparagus, egg yolks, dried plums, raisins, artichokes, spinach, and collard greens provide iron, which helps red blood cells carry oxygen throughout the body for energy.

Optimal Life Supplements

Vitamin C. Low levels have been correlated with reduced fat oxidation during exercise, which is also related to fatigue. Vitamin C can impact the synthesis of carnitine, an amino acid required for energy production from fatty acids. Low vitamin C status may play a role in the inability to shed pounds during weight-loss efforts.

Carnitine. A study showed that cancer-related fatigue dropped significantly in patients who had received intravenous carnitine supplementation. A significant increase in lean muscle mass was also noted for those who received the supplement. Oral carnitine supplementation can help, too.

CoQ_{10}. A small human study resulted in decreased fatigue sensation and improved physical performance during fatigue-inducing workload trials in those who took an oral coenzyme Q_{10} supplement.

Caution! *Caffeine and other herbal stimulants give only a quick fix when it comes to fatigue.*

WEIGHT LOSS

If you are overweight, losing even fifteen pounds can really make a difference in how you feel and perform. Obesity is one of the major contributors to sleep apnea, an insidious robber of energy!

Cynthia Sass's Tips for Losing Weight and Keeping It Off

Cynthia Sass, MPH, MA, RD, CSSD, is the coauthor of the Flat Belly Diet! Cookbook *and a contributing editor to* Shape *magazine.*

1. Nutrition for weight management is all about the big picture, including the quantity, quality, timing, balance, and enjoyment of the foods you eat. Vegetables; fruits; whole grains; lean proteins, including beans; healthy fats, including nuts; and fluids like water and tea are all important pieces of the weight-management puzzle.

2. Foods containing trans fats have been shown to increase body weight more than diets with a similar calorie level and add weight specifically in the midsection, the most dangerous place to carry excess body fat.

3. Artificial sweeteners work against people trying to lose weight. Animal research and my anecdotal experience as a practitioner have shown that artificial sweeteners can stoke a sweet tooth and snowball into a higher overall calorie intake.

4. Adequate sleep, stress management, social support, journaling, enjoyable physical activity (the kind you look forward to), realistic expectations, and patience are all key ingredients in the weight-loss recipe.

Feeding the Fire!

Caffeine. It's a quick fix that doesn't last long.

Dehydration equals fatigue.

Lighten up. Eating large, high-fat meals can slow down oxygen-carrying blood flow, causing "Thanksgiving dinner syndrome."

Skip the simple carbs. Eating a high-glycemic-load diet is strongly associated with fatigue.

ENERGIZING MENU PLAN

Day 1

Breakfast (520)
1 serving *Powerhouse Dried Plum Bars* (200) (page 343)
1 serving *Blackberry Smoothie* (320) (page 258)
1 cup green tea

Lunch (410)
1 serving *Roasted Vegetable and Sweet Swiss Panini* (250)
(page 333)
1 serving *Beanie-Greenie Brownies* (110) (page 309)
1 cup strawberries (50)
1½ cups water with lemon

Midday Snack (320)
1 serving *Zucchini-Cranberry Muffins* (190) (page 339)
1 serving *Apple-Soy Chai Latte* (130) (page 254)
1½ cups sparkling water with lime

Dinner (720)
4 ounces roast beef (or other meat or iron-fortified meat
replacer) (220)
1 serving *Warm Goat Cheese Salad with Hazelnuts and
Raspberries* (390) (page 295)
1 baked potato (110)
1½ cups water with lemon

Evening Snack (75)
½ cup carrot sticks (25)
2 tablespoons hummus (50)
1 cup decaffeinated green tea

Day 2

Breakfast (490)
1 serving *Soufflé Omelet with Balsamic Strawberries* (160)
(page 345)
1 serving *Nutty Good Millet Muffins* (240) (page 352)
1 cup skim milk (90)

Lunch (586)
1 serving *Asian Satay Skewers with Black Bean Sauce* (196)
(page 263)
½ serving *Quinoa Pilaf with Currants and Turmeric* (160)
(page 369)
1 serving *Quick Pumpkin Smoothie* (230) (page 256)

Midday Snack (290)
1 serving *Rosemary Nuts* (290) (page 269)
1 cup green tea

Dinner (574)
1 serving *Cocoa-Encrusted Salmon with Blueberries* (270)
(page 330)
1 serving *Roasted Autumn Vegetables in Sherry Sauce* (114)
(page 360)
½ cup brown rice (100)
1 cup skim milk (90)

Evening Snack (110)
1 serving *Beanie-Greenie Brownies* (110) (page 309)
1 cup decaffeinated green tea

Day 3

Breakfast (568)
1 serving *Triple-Grain Georgia Pecan Pancakes* (188) (page 346)
1 serving *Blackberry Smoothie* (320) (page 258)
1 apple (60)
1 cup tea or coffee

Lunch (529)
1 serving *Healthy Turkey Salad Pocket* (233) (page 335)
1 serving *Asparagus-Carrot Rolls* (210) (page 361)
1 cup strawberries (50)
1 serving *Watermelon Soda* (36) (page 253)
1 cup green tea

Midday Snack (130)
1 serving *Strawberry-Papaya Smoothie* (130) (page 255)

Dinner (586)
1 serving *Garlic Pipérade Soup* (150) (page 274)
1 serving *Chicken Thighs with Red Wine, Dried Plums, and Garlic* (310) (page 323)
1 steamed artichoke (90)
1 serving *Watermelon Soda* (36) (page 253)

Evening Snack (160)
1 serving *Raspberry-Yogurt Muffins* (160) (page 338)
1 cup chamomile tea

TARA GIDUS'S TOP TEN NUTRITION TIPS TO ENERGIZE YOUR GOLF GAME

Here's some great advice for the weekend warrior all the way up to Tiger Woods wannabees from Tara Gidus, MS, RD, CSSD, nutrition adviser and columnist for Golf Fitness Magazine.

1. *Stay well hydrated.* You need more water while exercising, especially on hot and humid days. Depending on the weather, you need to drink sixteen or more ounces of water per hour that you are on the course.

   Tara's faves: Water, flavored water, sports beverages.
2. *Eat while on the course.* Not eating will cause your blood sugar (glucose) to drop, leaving you fatigued and unfocused. A typical round of golf lasts more than three hours, so having a snack or two during play will keep you energized and focused.

   Tara's faves: Half a turkey sandwich with an apple.
3. *Eat before you go.* If you have an early tee time, it is sometimes difficult to think about eating breakfast. If you don't eat something before you play, you risk using muscle for energy instead of the food you would have eaten for breakfast. If a full breakfast is too much, just have something light and then bring snacks to eat on the course.

   Tara's faves: A bowl of whole grain cereal, milk, blueberries.
4. *Avoid foods high in sugar.* Drinking regular soda or eating candy on the course may give you a spike in glucose and energy, but it will be followed by a drop in energy level.

   Tara's faves: A low-fat beef or turkey jerky and a banana

will give you lasting energy as well as replenish sodium and potassium that you lose through sweat.

5. *Eat low-glycemic snacks.* Eating a snack with fiber and/or protein, as opposed to high-sugar or refined-flour snacks, before and during play will give you lasting energy. Think a handful of almonds instead of pretzels.

   Tara's faves: A handful of almonds or peanuts or a nutrition bar.

6. *Avoid alcohol and caffeine during play.* Alcohol is a depressant and it can significantly affect your concentration and coordination. If you care about the results of your game, save the drinking for later. Caffeine may slightly help performance, but too much can leave you jittery and unbalanced.

   Tara's faves: Drink water or caffeine-free iced tea during play instead of coffee and beer.

7. *Feed your brain to keep it happy.* If you had a bad game, instead of drowning your sorrows with a few drinks, have a meal that will provide your brain with food to make you feel good. Certain nutrients like vitamin D, folic acid, and omega-3s have been linked to improving mood and brain function.

   Tara's faves: Have a piece of salmon on a salad with a side of black bean soup.

8. *Restore your energy at the nineteenth hole.* The nineteenth hole is famous for lots of alcohol and fried food. Recovery with the right foods is vital to maintaining good energy and replenishing the muscles you just used on the course. Limit yourself to one drink and have a glass of water along with it to stay hydrated. Have a meal of a nice mix of complex carbs, some lean protein, and a little bit of fat.

> *Tara's faves: Lean roast beef with spinach and tomato in a whole wheat pita with a fruit cup.*

9. *Protect against injury.* The sun and exercise can do a body good, but they can cause your body to produce free radicals too, which attack your cells and lead to injury and disease. Eat fruits, vegetables, and whole grains before, during, and after your game to neutralize those free radicals and protect your cells.

> *Tara's faves: Have a smoothie with blueberries, strawberries, and raspberries. Add some wheat germ for even more antioxidant protection.*

10. *Reduce inflammation.* Omega-3s can not only protect the brain, but they can also hold back the inflammatory process. Omega-3 fats have been shown to reduce inflammation in the heart and all over the body.

> *Tara's faves: Have smoked salmon on a bagel for breakfast before you go out.*

SEXUAL/REPRODUCTIVE PERFORMANCE

ERECTILE DYSFUNCTION (ED)

On the Rise

Did you know... according to the Massachusetts Male Aging Study (1987–2004), overall prevalence of erectile dysfunction (ED) for a range of ages from forty to seventy was estimated at 44 percent? An astonishing 39 percent of forty-year-old men experienced ED on a regular basis in the study. Presently, with the rising rate of obesity, which is a significant risk factor for ED, many health experts surmise the current overall rate of ED to be over 50 percent, with a growing number of cases in men under the age of forty!

Optimal Food/Nutrient Highlights

Watermelon, cruciferous vegetables, arginine, citruline, carnitine.

What Is ED?

Healthy erectile function is universally considered by men to be a significant part of the "quality of life" equation. However, men often don't seek proper medical advice when their sex life doesn't measure up to expectations. This may be due in part to the lack of understanding of ED.

Erectile dysfunction can be defined as the inability to achieve or maintain an erection sufficient for satisfactory sexual performance. Achieving an erection involves both nervous system and vascular functions. Dysfunction in either of these areas can affect the ability to achieve an erection.

What Causes It?

Atherosclerotic disease. Recent studies show that ED in younger men may be an early warning sign of future hardening of the arteries. There are well-recognized risk factors for coronary artery disease, such as obesity, hypertension, and hypercholesterolemia, and all have been associated with ED. It is estimated that for 40 percent of men over the age of fifty, the primary cause of ED is related to atherosclerotic disease.

Metabolic syndrome/insulin resistance. There is a greater presence of metabolic syndrome and insulin resistance, which can contribute to atherosclerotic disease in those men diagnosed with ED.

Psychological causes. Depression, stress, poor self-esteem, and issues with one's body image can all be contributing factors to ED.

Hormonal (andropause and hypogonadism) imbalance. Levels of the hormone testosterone progressively decline as men age. Andropause is a condition where there is a decrease in one or more of the male sex hormones (androgens)—testosterone being one of the main androgens. As men age, they also produce more sex hormone–binding globulin (SHBG), which renders testosterone less effective. So a man could have low to normal testosterone levels, but if SHBG is elevated, it would be the same as having a deficiency of testosterone. This decrease in testosterone production can wreak havoc by negatively affecting body composition—resulting in diminished muscle size and strength, decreased bone mass, and increased adiposity (especially around the midsection)—while lowering energy levels and causing depression, poor cognition, and ultimately impaired sexual function.

There are a host of other causes of ED, including neurological and pharmacological complications (drug and cancer-treatment side effects), diabetes, disease of the penis itself, smoking, drug and alcohol use, and poor nutrition (the body needs to be fed well to perform!).

Optimal Life Foods

Lifestyle changes such as weight loss and increased physical activity have been associated with improvement in sexual function. The optimal life dietary foundation I espouse is very similar to a

Mediterranean type of diet, which has been shown to be beneficial for men battling ED. The cornerstones of both diets include olive oil, plenty of fruits and vegetables, whole grains, beans, nuts and seeds, low to moderate amounts of fish and poultry, low to moderate amounts of cheese and cultured dairy products, and moderate consumption of alcohol—preferably wine.

Arginine-rich foods. Arginine boosts nitric oxide in the bloodstream, which causes blood vessels to relax and fill with blood. Food sources of arginine include sesame seeds, almonds, peanuts, walnuts, Brazil nuts, coconut, dairy, soy, chickpeas, lean pork, beef, chicken, turkey, seafood, oats, wheat, and chocolate.

Citruline-rich foods. These increase production of the amino acid arginine. Citruline-rich foods include lean meats, fish, eggs, low-fat dairy, legumes, and watermelon (rind and flesh).

Cruciferous vegetables. Broccoli, cauliflower, kale, and Brussels sprouts contain indole-3-carbinol, which increases conversion of estradiol to a weaker form of estrogen. Higher estrogen levels in men have been associated with ED.

Optimal Life Supplements

L-arginine. Enhances nitric oxide production for more blood flow to where it counts.

L-carnitine. A double-blind study found those men who supplemented with carnitine had significant improvement in their ED.

Ginkgo biloba. Also improves vasodilation.

Korean ginseng. Sixty percent of participants in one study reported improvement in sexual function.

Caution!

Herbal Viagra. *Be careful of so-called natural alternatives, as they have been found to actually contain the drugs sildenafil (Viagra) and tadalafil (Cialis).*

Yohimbe. *There have been several studies on the use of the prescription medicine Yocon (yohimbine hydrochloride) for treating ED; Yocon is derived from the herb yohimbe. However, it is questionable if the herb produces the same effect as the medication. Yohimbe use has been associated with high blood pressure, headaches, dizziness, increased heart rate, and sleeplessness.*

Feeding the Fire!

A high-saturated-fat, high-trans-fat, high-cholesterol diet may contribute to atherosclerosis, limiting blood flow.

Grapefruit may cause ED medications to be overabsorbed. That may sound like a good thing at first, but in reality, it could be quite dangerous!

High alcohol intake activates the aromatase enzyme, which may also increase SHBG levels.

MALE SEXUAL PERFORMANCE MENU PLAN

Day 1

Breakfast (535)
1 serving *Capp-oat-ccino Delight* (340) (page 337)

1 cup light soy milk (110)

1½ cups diced watermelon (be sure to include the white part) (60)

1 teaspoon honey (25)

1 cup green tea

Lunch (476)

1 serving *Curried Chickpeas and Kale* (150) (page 370)

1 serving *Rosemary Nuts* (290) (page 269)

1 serving *Watermelon Soda* (36) (page 253)

Midday Snack (196)

1 serving *Asian Satay Skewers with Black Bean Sauce* (196) (page 263)

1½ cups sparkling water with lime

Dinner (605)

1 veggie-burger patty on a whole grain bun (280)

1 serving *Barley Salad with Edamame* (160) (page 287)

1 serving *Poached Pears* (165) (page 307)

1½ cups iced tea

Evening Snack (230)

1 serving *Quick Pumpkin Smoothie* (230) (page 256)

Day 2

Breakfast (450)

1 serving *Soufflé Omelet with Balsamic Strawberries* (160) (page 345)

1 slice whole grain toast with almond butter (180)

1 cup light soy milk (110)

Lunch (590)
1 serving *Watermelon and Feta Salad* (270) (page 294)
1 *Blackberry Smoothie* (320) (page 258)

Midday Snack (240)
1 serving *Beanie-Greenie Brownies* (110) (page 309)
1 serving *Apple-Soy Chai Latte* (130) (page 254)
1 cup green tea

Dinner (595)
1 serving *Cocoa-Encrusted Salmon with Blueberries* (270)
(page 330)
1 serving *Vegetable Pavé with Cauliflower Coulis* (60) (page 366)
1 whole grain roll (100)
1 serving *Poached Pears* (165) (page 307)
1½ cups water with lemon

Evening Snack (200)
1 serving *Apple-Soy Chai Latte* (130) (page 254)
1 serving *Cheese-and-Fruit Kebabs* (70) (page 272)

Day 3

Breakfast (400)
1 serving *Cherry–Chai Spice Granola* (240) (page 348)
1 cup mixed berries (50)
1 cup light soy milk (110)

Lunch (260)
1 serving *Tropical Fruit and Shrimp Gazpacho* (80) (page 279)
1 serving *Polenta Pizza* (180) (page 329)
1½ cups water with lemon

Midday Snack (383)
1 serving *Cherry Zinger Smoothie* (383) (page 256)

Dinner (546)
1 serving *Chicken Thighs with Red Wine, Dried Plums, and Garlic* (310) (page 323)
1 serving *Sicilian Broccoli Salad* (200) (page 291)
1 serving *Watermelon Soda* (36) (page 253)

Evening Snack (500)
1 serving *Summer Fruits Pie* (390) (page 315)
1 cup light soy milk (110)

Dave's Tips

1. Want more? Weigh less! There is an inverse relationship between body mass index and testosterone levels. Obesity depresses the production of testosterone.
2. Get physical. Men who started exercising in midlife experienced a 70 percent reduction in ED rates compared with those who weren't exercising.
3. Just say, "NO!" Eat more foods that encourage nitric oxide (NO) production, such as oats, almonds, grapes, seafood, and chocolate!

BENIGN PROSTATIC HYPERPLASIA (BPH)

It Is Our Destiny

Did you know... the estimated percentage of BPH in the United States is correlated with the age of the man? For example, 50 percent of men at the age of fifty and 80 percent of the men at age eighty have BPH. If a man lives long enough, odds are he will have a swollen prostate!

Optimal Food/Nutrient Highlights

Onions, garlic, yellow and green vegetables, soy, lycopene, green tea, alcohol, zinc, flavonoids, and beta-sitosterols.

What Is Benign Prostatic Hyperplasia?

Benign prostatic hyperplasia, also called benign prostatic hypertrophy, or BPH, aka "enlarged prostate," is a common affliction that men often suffer as they age. An average adult prostate is about the size of a walnut. But in BPH, there is an irregular enlargement. The prostate surrounds the urethra (where urine empties from the bladder), and as the prostate enlarges, urine flow becomes restricted. As the prostate continues to swell, stronger contractions of the bladder become necessary to push urine through the narrowed urethra, also causing a thickening of the bladder walls, which can reduce the bladder's capability of storing urine. Nocturnal urges and the frequent need for urination are common indicators of BPH.

What Causes It?

Although the cause of BPH is not well understood, it is often attributed in part to age, genetics, and age-related hormone changes.

Obesity. Obesity and central adiposity are major risk factors for BPH. A study in the *Journal of Clinical Endocrinology and Metabolism* found that men who were severely obese had a 3.5 times higher risk of developing BPH.

Poor glucose regulation. Both high and low blood glucose can affect insulin-like growth factors, which can contribute to prostate enlargement.

Hyperlipidemia. The presence of excess fat or lipids in the blood is a risk factor for both BPH and prostate cancer.

Chronic inflammation. Dietary factors such as low omega-3 fatty acid, polyunsaturated fat, and antioxidant intake allow for greater oxidative damage to the prostate gland.

Inactivity. In a study featured in *European Urology,* a review of eleven studies involving some 43,000 men found that those who exercised regularly had about a 25 percent reduced risk of BPH.

Optimal Life Foods

Beta-sitosterols. Soy, peanuts, and avocados are natural sources of this plant sterol. A review of the literature suggests that beta-sitosterols improve urinary symptoms and flow.

Zinc-rich foods. Dietary intake of zinc was associated with reduced risk in one study. Leading food sources of zinc include barley, chicken, oysters, crab, and wheat. Pumpkin seeds are rich in zinc and also rich in alanine, glycine, and glutamic acid, which are also believed to be protective against BPH.

Flavonoid-rich foods. Onions, apples, watermelon, green tea, and foods that are rich in plant estrogens such as cereals, grains, rye, soy, red clover, fruits, vegetables, flaxseed, peas, asparagus, plums, and pears are associated with a lower risk of BPH.

Onions and garlic. European studies showed an inverse relationship between eating foods in the onion and garlic family and the rate of BPH.

Yellow and green vegetables were also reported in a small case-control study to reduce risk of BPH.

Soy is a major source of the isoflavonoids daidzein and genistein. Both play a protective role against prostatic diseases.

Lycopene. Watermelon, papaya, pink grapefruit, and pink guava contain the plant chemical called lycopene (also found in tomatoes). Consumption of lycopene-rich foods is inversely related to the risk of developing BPH.

Green tea. Research has detected numerous compounds in green tea, including antioxidants, 5-alpha-reductase inhibitors, aromatase inhibitors, and tyrosine-specific protein kinase inhibitors. Polyphenols, commonly known as flavanols or catechins, have strong antioxidant activity and act as free-radical scavengers. One polyphenol in particular, epigallocatechin-3-gallate (EGCG), can modulate the production and effects of prostate-enlarging androgens and other hormones.

Alcohol. Numerous epidemiologic reports have generally shown a lower prevalence of BPH among alcohol consumers. Alcohol consumption in humans has been associated with increased serum estrogen and decreased levels of testosterone and SHBG, which may benefit BPH, but unfortunately does not help if you have erectile dysfunction. Moderation continues to be the key.

Optimal Life Supplements

Vitamin D. In preclinical studies, vitamin D_3 has been shown to reduce BPH cell growth.

Saw palmetto. A review study concluded that the herb saw palmetto provides slight improvement in urinary flow. A large study published in the *New England Journal of Medicine* in 2006 gave 225 men either saw palmetto or a placebo for a year and found no effect on self-reports of urinary symptoms or quality of life or on objective measures such as prostate size and urine-flow rate. It's possible that higher doses of the extract may provide better or more consistent results.

Pygeum africanum. A review of the literature confirmed that *Pygeum africanum,* a popular herb used to treat BPH, provides moderate relief from BPH-related symptoms.

Amino acids. The combination of glycine, alanine, and glutamic acid (200 mg of each daily) reduces urinary urgency, urinary frequency, and delayed initiation of flow.

Feeding the Fire!

Excess alcohol or fluid intake, especially at night, should be avoided.

Starchy foods like bread and highly refined cereals were positively associated with the risk of BPH in some European studies. However, no relation between cereal consumption and the risk of BPH was found in a case-control investigation from Greece. There may be a difference between the varieties of cereals consumed, specifically more coarse whole grain versus refined.

High-fat diets. Both high-polyunsaturated- and high-saturated-fat diets have been positively associated with the development of BPH.

Animal proteins. Studies have also found that high animal protein intake, especially in the presence of low vegetable intake, moderately increases BPH risk.

Dairy. Two studies found an increased risk of BPH associated with milk consumption, but a recent European population survey did not support previous findings. Additional studies are needed in milk-consuming populations to establish any significant causative role of milk in BPH.

ANTI-BPH MENU PLAN

Day 1

Breakfast (535)
1 serving *Capp-oat-ccino Delight* (340) (page 337)
1 cup light soy milk (110)
1½ cups diced watermelon (60)
1 teaspoon honey (25)
1 cup green tea

Lunch (479)
1 serving *Curried Chickpeas and Kale* (150) (page 370)
1 serving *Healthy Turkey Salad Pocket* (233) (page 335)
1 peach (60)
1 serving *Watermelon Soda* (36) (page 253)

Midday Snack (196)
1 serving *Asian Satay Skewers with Black Bean Sauce* (196) (page 263)
1½ cups sparkling water with lime

Dinner (560)
1 veggie-burger patty on a whole grain bun (280)
1 serving *Barley Salad with Edamame* (160) (page 287)
5 ounces red wine (optional) (120)

Evening Snack (230)
1 serving *Chilean Fruit Guacamole* (100) (page 259)
1 serving *Apple-Soy Chai Latte* (130) (page 254)

Day 2

Breakfast (450)
1 serving *Soufflé Omelet with Balsamic Strawberries* (160)
(page 345)
1 slice whole grain toast with almond butter (180)
1 cup light soy milk (110)

Lunch (590)
1 serving *Watermelon and Feta Salad* (270) (page 294)
1 serving *Blackberry Smoothie* (320) (page 258)

Midday Snack (110)
1 serving *Beanie-Greenie Brownies* (110) (page 309)
1 cup green tea

Dinner (720)
1 serving *Cocoa-Encrusted Salmon with Blueberries* (270)
(page 330)
1 serving *Avocado-Fennel Citrus Salad* (120) (page 285)
1 serving *Japanese-Style Vegetable Fried Rice* (230)
(page 355)
1 whole grain roll (100)
$1\frac{1}{2}$ cups water with lemon

Evening Snack (80)
2 servings *Kale Balls* (80) (page 262)
1 cup decaffeinated green tea

Day 3

Breakfast (370)
1 serving *Cherry–Chai Spice Granola* (240) (page 348)
1 serving *Strawberry-Papaya Smoothie* (130) (page 255)

Lunch (550)
1 serving *Curried Chicken-Banana-Yam Soup* (280) (page 280)
1 serving *Watermelon and Feta Salad* (270) (page 294)
1½ cups water with lemon

Midday Snack (130)
1 serving *Spicy Biscotti* (130) (page 311)
1 cup green tea

Dinner (586)
4 ounces baked chicken tenders with 1 serving *Raspberry Salsa* (page 299) (250)
1 serving *Sicilian Broccoli Salad* (200) (page 291)
½ cup brown rice (100)
1 serving *Watermelon Soda* (36) (page 253)

Evening Snack (390)
1 serving *Summer Fruits Pie* (390) (page 315)
1 cup decaffeinated green tea

Dave's Tips

1. Kick the habit. As if you need another reason to quit smoking, research has found an elevated risk of BPH among heavy smokers.
2. Walk it off. Even moderate physical activity such as walking has been found to be inversely associated with total BPH.

3. Go with the flow. Avoid delaying urination and be careful about your fluid intake by limiting the amount of fluid consumed at any one time and avoiding beverages after 7 P.M.

4. Go green. Try having green tea instead of your daily cup of coffee.

5. Be a soy boy! Try substituting sources of soy protein (which may reduce the risk of BPH) for animal products like red meat, eggs, and chicken (which may contribute to an increased risk).

6. Fight vampires (and BPH) with garlic! Try using the deliciously potent ingredient in salad dressings, sandwiches, and pasta dishes. You can even spread roasted garlic directly on some crusty bread.

INFERTILITY

Inconceivable

Did you know... infertility affects approximately 6.1 million individuals throughout the United States? Although infertility is often blamed on women, each gender shares an equal third of the responsibility, with the remaining third being attributed to reasons unknown.

Optimal Food/Nutrient Highlights

Salmon, walnuts, red wine, Concord grapes, chocolate, plant sterols, zinc, folate, calcium.

What Is Infertility?

Infertility is a condition of the reproductive system that impairs the conception of children. The diagnosis of infertility is usually given to couples who have been attempting to conceive for at least one year without success. Infertility can occur in any number of stages during conception and pregnancy.

What Causes It?

Decreased numbers and quality of sperm. Azoospermia is a condition where no sperm cells are produced, and oligospermia is where very few sperm cells are produced. Sperm cells can also become malformed or die prematurely before reaching the egg. Lifestyle factors negatively affecting sperm production and sexual performance include smoking; drug and alcohol abuse; exposure to toxins such as chemicals, pesticides, and lead; sexually transmitted diseases (STDs); diabetes; genetic diseases; viruses; mumps; prostatitis; testicular disease or injury; and medications (antihypertensives, diuretics, and beta-blockers).

Ovulation disorders. Oligo-ovulation (irregular egg production) and anovulation (lack of egg production) are the most common female infertility factors. The ovaries' ability to produce eggs declines with age and with certain medical conditions.

Polycystic ovary syndrome. PCOS affects 5 to 10 percent of women of reproductive age and is characterized by excess androgen production, polycystic ovaries, acne, and infrequent or lack of menses. Insulin resistance, which is characteristic of a condition called metabolic syndrome that also involves central adiposity and obesity, is frequently seen in women diagnosed with PCOS. Insulin resistance increases androgen production.

Eating disorders, excessive exercise, and hypothalamic amenorrhea. These conditions negatively affect both body composition and nutrition status and have been associated with abnormal levels of the hormone leptin, which in turn has been found to affect fertility.

Blocked fallopian tubes. Pelvic inflammatory disease and endometriosis are common causes of blocked fallopian tubes.

Inability of the embryo to implant in the uterus. Birth defects otherwise known as congenital anomalies can alter the structure of the uterus, making it difficult for the embryo to implant.

Embryo viability. Fibroids in the uterus are also associated with repeated miscarriages. A diet lacking in adequate antioxidants can create an environment of oxidative stress that not only negatively influences conception, but also diminishes chances for sustaining a pregnancy.

Optimal Life Foods

Optimal life diet. A base diet of colorful fruits and vegetables, whole grains, lean meats, beans and plant-based proteins, low-fat dairy products, nuts, seeds, and quality oils nourishes the body best for reproduction. A Spanish study found that healthy male subjects who had higher sperm quality consumed adequate levels of high-fiber-containing carbohydrates, folate, and antioxidants, including vitamin C and lycopene. These subjects also had lower intakes of proteins and total fat compared with men presenting with poor sperm quality.

Angela Grassi's Top Ten Food Tips for Treating PCOS

Angela Grassi, MS, RD, LDN, is the author of The PCOS Workbook *and* The Dietitian's Guide to Polycystic Ovary

Syndrome *and one of the leading authorities on dietary approaches to treating PCOS-related infertility.*

1. *Salmon (or other fatty-type fish).* Eat fatty fish, rich in omega-3 fats, to reduce inflammation and lipid levels and to improve insulin resistance, skin, and even mood.

2. *Walnuts and almonds* contain omega-3 and monounsaturated, heart-healthy fats.

3. *Whole grains* contain vitamins, minerals, and fiber to reduce cholesterol, inflammation, and insulin and to improve ovulation.

4. *Focus on fruits,* as they contain important vitamins, minerals, fiber, and antioxidants to reduce insulin, cholesterol, and inflammation.

5. *Vary your vegetables.* Improve insulin resistance, reduce lipid levels, and prevent cancer by eating a wide array of veggies.

6. *Lean on proteins.* Studies show that women who eat mostly lean protein foods like skinless poultry and plant-based proteins have better fertility.

7. *Dairy products.* Milk and yogurt are rich sources of vitamin D, which studies show can help reduce insulin. For weight management, choose low-fat dairy, which has less fat and calories. But if you're trying to get pregnant, one or two servings of whole-fat dairy can improve fertility.

8. *Plant sterols.* Naturally found in vegetable oils, nuts, and whole grains, plant sterols are now being added to numerous foods like juice, granola bars, mayonnaise, margarines, milk, and even multivitamins. Adding plant sterols to your diet is one of the simplest ways to lower your cholesterol.

9. *Dark chocolate* is rich in flavanols, which, studies show, can reduce inflammation.

10. *Red wine and Concord grape juice* are both rich in polyphenols and antioxidants. Grape juice may be the preferred option for

protection against cardiovascular disease and inflammation when you are trying to get pregnant.

Other Foods That Support Fertility

Essential fatty acids help promote ovulation. Excellent sources include fatty fish such as salmon, mackerel, sardines, and tuna; nuts like walnuts and almonds, and seeds like flax and pumpkin seed; eggs; soy; and olive and canola oil.

Zinc-rich foods. Oysters, crab, pork, beef, chicken, and turkey help in sperm and testosterone production in men, and in ovulation and fertility in women. Studies indicate that deficiencies in zinc impede both male and female fertility.

Folate. This B vitamin helps reduce risk of neural tube birth defects. Food sources include spinach and other dark green leafy vegetables, citrus fruits, nuts, legumes, whole grains, and fortified breads and cereals.

Calcium. Women should get in at least 1,000 mg of calcium (three 8-ounce glasses of skim milk) a day if they are considering getting pregnant. Calcium may be obtained from natural sources such as cottage cheese, low-fat yogurt, canned salmon, sardines, and cheese.

Optimal Life Supplements

Angela's Top Ten Supplement Tips for Treating PCOS

1. *Inositol* helps improve insulin sensitivity and ovulation.
2. *Magnesium* helps reduce insulin, glucose, cholesterol, blood pressure, and overall risk of metabolic syndrome.

3. *Cinnamon* can lower insulin and cholesterol.

4. *Chromium* lowers insulin and glucose.

5. *Fish oil* reduces triglycerides, insulin, and inflammation, and improves skin and mood.

6. *Alpha-lipoic acid* improves insulin resistance.

7. *Vitamin D* decreases insulin and helps with ovulation.

8. *Saw palmetto* lowers testosterone and reduces inflammation.

9. *Biotin* keeps skin and hair healthy and improves insulin resistance.

10. *N-acetyl cysteine* improves insulin sensitivity.

Research has shown that a multivitamin and mineral supplement can improve chances of conception. Start on a good prenatal formula before trying to conceive. Consult with a registered dietitian who specializes in fertility, your pharmacist, or your doctor for recommendations.

Caution! *Avoid caffeinated supplements. Apart from prenatal formulas, the safety of many dietary supplements in relationship to pregnancy is unknown. Some herbal formulas are known to increase risk of miscarriage. Consult with a registered dietitian, your pharmacist, or your doctor before taking any supplement.*

Feeding the Fire!

Alcohol. Although many babies have been conceived when alcohol has been consumed, it is a good idea to limit or avoid alcohol, as it may interfere with conception. Couples who are having difficulty in conceiving in particular should avoid all alcohol.

Caffeinated foods, beverages, and over-the-counter medicines. Some studies have linked caffeine to infertility, but more recent ones indicate that moderate consumption, up to about three 8-ounce cups of brewed coffee a day—or below 300 mg—should be fine. More than 300 mg of caffeine per day may reduce fertility by 27 percent!

Fad diets. Adequate body fat is needed for hormone production. Although many women having difficulties conceiving are overweight or obese, being too thin can work against conception, too!

FERTILITY MENU PLAN

This menu plan is geared a bit more to women, especially those who may be experiencing PCOS. It includes more of Angela's recommendations.

Day 1

Breakfast (365)
1 cup flaxseed cereal flakes (190)
1 cup skim milk (90)
1 kiwi (60)
1 teaspoon honey (25)
1 cup green tea

Lunch (640)
2 servings *Kale Balls* (80) (page 262)
1 serving *Sardine Salad / Dip* (page 265) with ½ whole wheat pita cut into triangles (420)
1 cup strawberries (50)
1 cup skim milk (90)

Midday Snack (220)
1 serving *Chilean Fruit Guacamole* (100) (page 259)
12 fat-free corn chips (120)
1½ cups sparkling water with lime

Dinner (580)
4 ounces rotisserie chicken (220)
1 whole grain roll with plant sterol margarine (150)
1 cup steamed Brussels sprouts (60)
2 cups spinach salad with assorted veggies and *Yogurt Sauce* dressing (page 305) (80)
½ cup Concord grape juice (70)

Evening Snack (260)
1 serving *Spicy Biscotti* (130) (page 311)
1 cup *Apple-Soy Chai Latte* (130) (page 254)

Day 2

Breakfast (450)
1 serving *Soufflé Omelet with Balsamic Strawberries* (160) (page 345)
1 whole grain English muffin with plant sterol margarine (200)
1 cup skim milk (90)

Lunch (540)
1 serving *Roasted Vegetable and Sweet Swiss Panini* (250) (page 333)
1 serving *Rosemary Nuts* (290) (page 269)
1½ cups water with lemon

Midday Snack (240)
1 serving *Nutty Good Millet Muffins* (240) (page 352)
1 cup green tea

Dinner (700)
1 serving *Cocoa-Encrusted Salmon with Blueberries* (270)
(page 330)
1 serving *Roasted Root Vegetables* (240) (page 365)
1 whole grain roll (100)
1 cup skim milk (90)

Evening Snack (110)
1 serving *Beanie-Greenie Brownies* (110) (page 309)
1 cup decaffeinated green tea

Day 3

Breakfast (310)
1 serving *Powerhouse Dried Plum Bars* (200) (page 343)
4 ounces high-probiotic yogurt (110)
1 cup green tea

Lunch (475)
1 serving *Tropical Fruit and Shrimp Gazpacho* (80) (page 279)
1 serving *Raw Kale Salad with Lemon-Honey Vinaigrette* (260)
(page 296)
1 whole grain roll with plant sterol margarine (150)
1½ cups water with lemon

Midday Snack (230)
1 serving *Quick Pumpkin Smoothie* (230) (page 256)

Dinner (735)
1 serving *Chicken Thighs with Red Wine, Dried Plums, and
Garlic* (310) (page 323)
1 serving *Sicilian Broccoli Salad* (200) (page 291)
½ cup brown rice with plant sterol margarine (135)
1 cup skim milk (90)

Evening Snack (250)
1 serving *Raspberry-Yogurt Muffins* (160) (page 338)
1 cup skim milk (90)

FEMALE LIBIDO

Lost That Lovin' Feeling?

Did you know... men and women have been pursuing ways to enhance their love lives for the past 5,000 years? And recent studies
indicate that approximately 40 percent of women aged eighteen to
fifty-nine have significant complaints about their sex lives!

Optimal Food/Nutrient Highlights

Asparagus, avocados, turkey, soy, arginine.

What Is Libido?

Simply put, *libido* means "sex drive." According to *Merriam-
Webster's Collegiate Dictionary,* libido is an "instinctual psychic

energy that...is derived from primitive biological urges (as for sexual pleasure or self-preservation) and that is expressed in conscious activity."

What Causes Libido to Be Low?

Sex drive will vary greatly throughout life. Much of it can be attributed to our state of mind, but there can also be underlying medical conditions that negatively affect libido. The most common negative influences on libido are

- Pregnancy and breast-feeding
- Troubled relationships
- Major life changes
- Illness
- Fatigue and stress
- Psychological issues such as poor body image and lack of intimacy
- Pain during sex or sexual dysfunction
- Surgery
- Alcohol and side effects of medications such as antihypertensives, antidepressants, and antihistamines
- Hormonal changes that result in irregular periods, breast tenderness, and vaginal dryness.

Optimal Life Foods

Arginine helps produce nitric oxide, which relaxes blood vessels to allow more blood flow to the sex organs. Arginine-rich foods include soy, peanuts, crab, shrimp, lobster, spinach, spirulina (seaweed), sesame, turkey, sunflower seeds, chicken, and eggs. Other foods that raise nitric oxide include Concord grapes, oats, pomegranates, and olive oil.

Asparagus is rich in both folate and a plant substance called protodioscin, which has been known to enhance nitric oxide.

Avocados contain high levels of folic acid.

Optimal Life Supplements

ArginMax (Panax ginseng, L-arginine, ginkgo biloba, damiana, and vitamins/minerals). A double-blind study of women of various ages showed the supplement enhanced libido most notably in postmenopausal women.

Muira puama and ginkgo biloba are two herbs that were combined in a study investigating alternatives to prescription medications for sexual dysfunction in over 200 women. Sixty-five percent reported improvement in libido after taking the supplement.

Maca is a vegetable grown throughout South America but predominately in the Andes region. In a study of women who experienced sexual dysfunction while on SSRI antidepressants, those who supplemented with maca reported significant improvement in libido.

Caution! *Beware of herbal formulas claiming to enhance your love life! Some have been found to contain medications that could be potentially harmful.*

Feeding the Fire!

Smoking. Nicotine was found to significantly impair sexual arousal in women.

High-cholesterol, high-saturated-fat, and high-trans-fat diets can set up roadblocks on the streets of desire.

FEMALE LIBIDO MENU PLAN

Day 1

Breakfast (535)
1 serving *Capp-oat-ccino Delight* (340) (page 337)
1 cup light soy milk (110)
1½ cups diced watermelon (60)
1 teaspoon honey (25)
1 cup green tea

Lunch (519)
1 serving *Curried Chickpeas and Kale* (150) (page 370)
1 serving *Healthy Turkey Salad Pocket* (233) (page 335)
1 cup Concord grapes (100)
1 serving *Watermelon Soda* (36) (page 253)

Midday Snack (196)
1 serving *Asian Satay Skewers with Black Bean Sauce* (196)
(page 263)
1½ cups sparkling water with lime

Dinner (560)
1 veggie-burger patty on a whole grain bun (280)
1 serving *Barley Salad with Edamame* (160) (page 287)
5 ounces red wine (optional) (120)

Evening Snack (255)
½ cup carrot sticks (25)
1 serving *Chilean Fruit Guacamole* (100) (page 259)
1 serving *Apple-Soy Chai Latte* (130) (page 254)

Day 2

Breakfast (450)
1 serving *Soufflé Omelet with Balsamic Strawberries* (160)
(page 345)
1 slice whole grain toast with almond butter (180)
1 cup light soy milk (110)

Lunch (670)
1 small lobster tail, or crabmeat or shrimp, to top 1 serving
Avocado-Fennel Citrus Salad (page 285) (350)
1 serving *Blackberry Smoothie* (320) (page 258)

Midday Snack (240)
1 serving *Beanie-Greenie Brownies* (110) (page 309)
1 serving *Apple-Soy Chai Latte* (130) (page 254)
1 cup green tea

Dinner (450)
1 serving *Mediterranean Grilled Mackerel or Bluefish* (250)
(page 321)
1 serving *Asparagus-Sesame Stir-Fry* (100) (page 362)
1 whole grain roll (100)
1½ cups water with lemon

Evening Snack (216)
1 serving *Crumb-Topped Georgia Pecan and Cherry Cereal
Bars* (216) (page 341)
1 cup decaffeinated green tea

Day 3

Breakfast (400)
1 serving *Cherry–Chai Spice Granola* (240) (page 348)
½ cup pomegranate juice (70)
1 cup skim milk (90)

Lunch (390)
1 serving *Tropical Fruit and Shrimp Gazpacho* (80)
(page 279)
1 serving *Polenta Pizza* (180) (page 329)
1 serving *Apple-Soy Chai Latte* (130) (page 254)
1½ cups water with lemon

Midday Snack (225)
½ whole grain bagel (115)
1 serving *Super Fruit Relish* (225) (page 304)

Dinner (766)
1 serving *Potato-Corn Chowder* (220) (page 273)
1 serving *Chicken Thighs with Red Wine, Dried Plums, and
Garlic* (310) (page 323)
1 serving *Sicilian Broccoli Salad* (200) (page 291)
1 serving *Watermelon Soda* (36) (page 253)

Evening Snack (260)
1 serving *Pan-Cooked Apples and Pears in Grape Juice* (150)
(page 313)
1 cup light soy milk (110)

Dave's Tips

1. Pursue a healthy lifestyle. It's all connected. Increasing blood flow throughout the entire body helps nourish every part. A healthy lifestyle that includes the optimal life diet along with exercise and proper rest can really make a big difference in libido.
2. Regular exercise that includes both aerobic activity and strength training improves both physical and mental performance. Kegel exercises can also strengthen pelvic muscles.
3. Eat happy! Having a more positive and happy outlook and not being a worrywart are important to creating sexual desire. Not only should you focus on foods that stoke the furnace of desire because of their nutritional value, but you should take advantage of the mere act of dining with your partner to help get you both in a romantic mood. Do something different—go on a picnic, have a candlelit dinner, or have dinner in bed together!

MENOPAUSE

You're on Fire!

Did you know . . . some women's skin temperature can rise six degrees while they're having a hot flash?

Optimal Food/Nutrient Highlights

Dairy, vitamin D, soy, beans, fatty fish, flaxseed.

What Is Menopause?

Menopause means "end of menstruation." To be "perimenopausal" is to be in the transitional stage between the childbearing years and the cessation of menses and egg production. To be in menopause requires the complete absence of menstruation for a year.

At the same time, the hormone estrogen diminishes, and with that, hot flashes often begin, cognition can decline, and there is an increased risk of heart disease and osteoporosis. The average age of menopause is fifty-one, but it may start for women in their late thirties and early forties. Other symptoms of perimenopause/menopause include disruption of sleep and loss of energy, hormonal changes, irregular periods, decreased fertility, vaginal dryness, increased abdominal fat, thinning of hair, loss of breast fullness, and weight gain.

What Causes It?

Menopause is a natural part of the aging process, though women can be "thrown into" menopause early for several reasons, including hysterectomy, chemotherapy and radiation, autoimmune disorders, viral infections, and genetics.

Optimal Life Foods

Calcium- and vitamin D–rich foods are crucial for bone health. (See "Optimal Life Foods" for osteoporosis, on page 212.)

Hot Flashes, Night Sweats, and Vaginal Dryness

Phytoestrogens. Plant-based foods, especially ones that contain natural plant estrogens such as isoflavones and lignans, work in the body like a weak form of estrogen. These foods may help relieve menopause symptoms such as hot flashes, night sweats, and vaginal dryness. Besides soybeans and soy products such as tofu, tempeh, and soy milk, other significant sources of phytoestrogens include flaxseed, garlic, multigrain cereal and bread, chickpeas, licorice, black beans, sage, and pistachios.

Optimal Life Supplements

Omega-3 fats. Depression is yet another common symptom of menopause. In a study conducted by researchers at Laval University's Faculty of Medicine, in Quebec, women who were menopausal and mildly depressed were given either an omega-3 supplement of fish oil or a placebo. The fish oil group reported fewer depressive symptoms than the placebo group.

Black cohosh. While research on the effectiveness of this herb may be somewhat mixed, many of my patients have reported great results. Several women have told me that they "can't live without it" when it comes to controlling hot flashes and vaginal dryness.

Soy isoflavones are plant compounds that have a similar chemical structure to human estrogens. Genistein and daidzein are considered to be the most potent estrogens of the phytoestrogens found to help cognition, diminish hot flashes, and improve bone health.

Caution! *Wild yam (*Dioscorea villosa*) is a popular natural alternative for hot flashes. Unfortunately, an animal study linked its use with fibrosis of the kidney cells and inflammation in livers of rats after only twenty-eight days of being on this supplement.*

Feeding the Fire!

Some women report that spicy foods, caffeine, and alcohol exacerbate hot flashes.

MENOPAUSE MENU PLAN

Day 1

Breakfast (475)
1 cup flaxseed cereal flakes (190)
1 cup skim milk (90)
5 dried plums (110)
½ cup orange juice (calcium and vitamin D fortified) (60)
1 teaspoon honey (25)
1 cup green tea

Lunch (460)
1 serving *Roasted Vegetable and Sweet Swiss Panini* (250)
(page 333)
1 ounce pistachios (160)
1 cup strawberries (50)
1½ cups water with lemon

Midday Snack (220)
1 serving *Chilean Fruit Guacamole* (100) (page 259)
12 fat-free corn chips (120)
1½ cups sparkling water with lime

Dinner (546)
1 serving *Garlic Pipérade Soup* (150) (page 274)

1 serving *Asian Satay Skewers with Black Bean Sauce* (196)
(page 263)
2 cups spinach salad with assorted veggies and *Yogurt Sauce*
dressing (page 305) (80)
5 ounces red wine (optional) (120)

Evening Snack (205)
½ cup carrot sticks (25)
2 tablespoons hummus (50)
1 serving *Apple-Soy Chai Latte* (130) (page 254)

Day 2

Breakfast (510)
1 serving *Soufflé Omelet with Balsamic Strawberries* (160)
(page 345)
1 whole grain bagel (230)
1 serving *Fruit and Walnut Jam Conserve* (30) (page 302)
1 cup skim milk (90)

Lunch (530)
1 serving *Blackberry Smoothie* (320) (page 258)
1 serving *Avocado-Fennel Citrus Salad* (120) (page 285)
1 cup skim milk (90)

Midday Snack (290)
1 serving *Rosemary Nuts* (290) (page 269)
1 cup green tea

Dinner (574)
1 serving *Cocoa-Encrusted Salmon with Blueberries* (270)
(page 330)

1 serving *Roasted Autumn Vegetables in Sherry Sauce* (114)
(page 360)
1 whole grain roll (100)
1 cup skim milk (90)

Evening Snack (140)
1 serving *Christine's Baked Custard* (140) (page 308)
1 cup decaffeinated green tea

Day 3

Breakfast (508)
1 serving *Triple-Grain Georgia Pecan Pancakes* (188)
(page 346)
½ cup hash browns (120)
1 cup diced mango (110)
1 cup skim milk (90)

Lunch (430)
1 serving *Tropical Fruit and Shrimp Gazpacho* (80) (page 279)
1 serving *Raw Kale Salad with Lemon-Honey Vinaigrette* (260)
(page 296)
1 cup skim milk (90)
1½ cups water with lemon

Midday Snack (130)
1 serving *Strawberry-Papaya Smoothie* (130) (page 255)

Dinner (696)
1 serving *Chicken Thighs with Red Wine, Dried Plums, and
Garlic* (310) (page 323)
1 serving *Curried Chickpeas and Kale* (150) (page 370)

1 serving *Sicilian Broccoli Salad* (200) (page 291)
1 serving *Watermelon Soda* (36) (page 253)

Evening Snack (140)
1 serving *Christine's Baked Custard* (140) (page 308)
1 cup decaffeinated green tea

Dave's Tips

1. Working out regularly improves mood, eases pain and hot flashes, reduces risk of heart disease, and improves bone density.
2. Manage cholesterol and weight, which often rise during menopause. Losing 10 percent of your body weight can have a significant effect on reducing high cholesterol, a major risk for heart disease.
3. Managing stress through meditation, yoga, and relaxation techniques often reduces hot flashes.
4. Smoking and menopause don't mix, so quit! You are at even greater risk of osteoporosis and heart disease when you mix the two!
5. Get out of the kitchen! Avoid these triggers of hot flashes: Hot anything! Food, showers, saunas, sun, baths, tubs...you get the idea; caffeine and alcohol; George Clooney or Brad Pitt.

PART 5

CHECK YOUR PLUMBING

CONSTIPATION/DIVERTICULAR DISEASE

The Simple Things in Life...

Did you know... constipation is the most common digestive complaint in the United States? Millions of Americans, mostly over the age of sixty-five, are bothered enough from constipation to warrant more than 2.5 million physician visits a year. An additional $725 million are spent on laxative products.

Optimal Food/Nutrient Highlights

Whole grains, fresh and dried fruits, nuts and seeds, beans, fiber, probiotics and prebiotics, fluids.

What Are Constipation and Diverticular Disease?

Constipation is generally the precursor to diverticular disease, and the treatment of the two is quite similar.

Constipation occurs when the colon absorbs too much water, or if the normal contractions of the muscles in the bowel, also known as peristalsis, are too slow or sluggish. As a result, stools become hard and dry. The American College of Gastroenterology Chronic Constipation Task Force has defined chronic constipation as a disorder with at least three months of unsatisfactory bowel movements. "Unsatisfactory" includes infrequent stools (less than three times per week) and difficult stool passage (straining, a sense of difficulty passing stool, hard or lumpy stools, prolonged time to pass stool, or need for manual maneuvers to pass stool).

Many people think that they are experiencing constipation if they don't have a bowel movement every day. Yet stool elimination varies from individual to individual. Some people may "go" several times a day, others only a few times a week. Most constipation isn't in and of itself serious. The majority of problems are due to straining, which can lead to hemorrhoids and rectal prolapse. Dry and hard stools can also cause tearing in the skin around the anus.

Diverticular disease. Diverticula are fingerlike projections that protrude from the wall of the bowel. Straining to evacuate leads to increased pressure within the bowel and over time can cause diverticula to form (diverticulosis). Most who have diverticulosis don't even know it until one of the pouches becomes inflamed—a very painful condition known as diverticulitis. Approximately 60 percent of those who live in Westernized cultures and are over the age of sixty will develop diverticulosis. And for those fortunate to make it past the age of eighty-five, the percentage increases to 70 percent. About 25 percent of those who have diverticulosis will eventually have diverticulitis.

Signs and symptoms of diverticulitis include fever, abdominal pain (the most common symptom on examination is tenderness in the lower left side of the abdomen), gastrointestinal bleeding, and elevated white blood cell count.

Complications of diverticular disease can include bleeding, abscess, obstruction, fistula, and perforation. If diverticulosis is suspected, your doctor may prescribe radiologic tests, such as an ultrasound and computerized tomography (CT) scan, and a colonoscopy.

What Causes Constipation?

Chronic constipation can be due to a variety of factors, but most often, it can be attributed to a poor diet that lacks adequate fiber and hydration, accompanied by insufficient exercise. However, constipation can also be the side effect of a medication, or even more telling, of an underlying medical condition. The most common medical conditions include neurological disorders, metabolic and endocrine disorders, stroke, diabetes, hypothyroidism, colon and rectum adhesions, irritable bowel syndrome, and diverticulitis. Medications such as narcotics, antidepressants, iron supplements, and diuretics may also cause chronic constipation.

Beyond a poor diet, other contributing causes include ignoring the urge to have a bowel movement, changes in life or routine (e.g., pregnancy, travel), lack of physical activity, and stress.

Optimal Life Foods

High-fiber foods. Fiber works naturally to add bulk and water to stools so they can pass more easily through the intestines. In a review of twenty studies, eighteen of them made a clear connection between fiber and the relief of constipation. One of the studies that looked at over 62,000 women and evaluated the association between dietary fiber intake and constipation found that those who had the highest intake of dietary fiber (greater than twenty grams per day) were less likely to experience constipation than those who consumed less than seven grams a day. And those women who consumed over twenty grams of fiber who were also physically active had a threefold less prevalence of constipation than those who were following a low-fiber diet and did not exercise.

Unfortunately, Americans on average consume only five to fourteen grams of fiber a day. This falls woefully short of the 2005 *Dietary Guidelines for Americans* recommendation of thirty-five grams a day. Ideally, a combination of soluble- and insoluble-fiber food sources works best to promote digestive health. Those optimal life foods richest in a variety of fiber types are

- Whole grains such as teff, wheat, wheat bran, oats, barley, rye, millet, buckwheat, spelt, sorghum, and corn.
- Fresh and dried fruits, including apples, oranges, pears, strawberries, apricots, dried plums, dates, figs, raisins, cranberries, currants, kiwis, grapes, grapefruit, peaches, raspberries, blackberries, passion fruit, guavas, avocados, mangoes, blueberries, and persimmons.
- Nuts and seeds, including flaxseeds, sesame seeds, almonds, pecans, pistachios, and hazelnuts.
- Vegetables such as dried beans (e.g., navy, kidney, and pinto beans), carob, soybeans, lentils, carrots, broccoli, beets, artichokes, cauliflower, fennel, pumpkin, spinach, potatoes, and sweet potatoes.

Not everyone who suffers from constipation will see a benefit from eating a high-fiber diet. This may be because they don't consume enough fluids to meet the demands of higher fiber intake.

Fiber for Diverticulosis

A high-fiber diet, up to forty-five grams a day, is recommended. Slowly increase fiber in the diet up to this level to avoid discomfort.

Probiotics and Prebiotics

Probiotic foods include those that are naturally fermented and rich in friendly bacteria such as yogurt, kefir, sauerkraut, kimchi, and unpasteurized miso, all of which can help keep you running smoothly. Probiotics promote more frequent bowel evacuation, softer stools, and reduced strain.

Prebiotics are components found in foods that can't be broken down in the stomach and are fermentable in the large intestine. Prebiotics help create a favorable environment for probiotics to take hold. Food sources include whole grains, bananas, honey, agave, onions and leeks, and artichokes.

Fluids

As you increase your daily fiber, you want to increase your fluids as well. On average, six to eight cups of water a day will meet the needs of most people.

Optimal Life Supplements

Wheat bran. One heaping tablespoon on breakfast cereal or mixed into other foods is a great way to get fiber.

Ground flaxseeds. One to two tablespoons per day. Flax can be added to breakfast cereal, juice, or other foods. (For maximum freshness, buy the whole seeds and grind them as needed in a coffee grinder or blender.)

Fiber supplements (aka "bulking agents") include oat bran; psyllium (one brand: Metamucil); polycarbophil (one brand: FiberCon); and methylcellulose (one brand: Citrucel). The good news is that bulk-forming laxatives can be used every day without causing dependence.

Tryphala is a mixture of three fruits from India from the Ayurvedic tradition; it is available in capsule form at health food stores.

Magnesium glycinate may also be helpful for chronic constipation.

Probiotics help establish a good population of friendly bacteria in the colon that aids in digestion.

Caution! *Ferrous sulfate, a commonly found form of iron, has often been attributed to contributing to constipation and causing black and tarry stools. Preferable forms of iron may include ferrous bisglycinate capsules and Floradix liquid, which both can be obtained at most health food stores.*

Feeding the Fire!

Diets high in the following foods may be problematic for those experiencing chronic constipation:

Cheese, eggs, meats.

Refined and processed foods.

Caffeine-containing beverages such as coffee and cola drinks. A study showed that coffee intake of more than six cups a day is associated with a slightly increased risk of constipation. However, low to moderate consumption is associated with a reduced risk of constipation.

Alcohol can contribute to dehydration and decreased motility of the bowel.

Not consuming adequate calories, for example, in patients with anorexia nervosa, can cause constipation.

Feeding the Fire (Diverticular Disease)!

Nuts, seeds, popcorn, and hulls. Many in the medical profession believe that seeds may become lodged in the diverticula, causing inflammation. Not all seeds are of concern—those found in tomatoes, zucchini, cucumbers, strawberries, and raspberries, as well as poppy seeds, are generally considered harmless. Although there isn't enough scientific data for doctors to recommend with 100 percent confidence that their patients should avoid these foods, many gastroenterologists still steer their patients away from them. My clinical observation has been that seeds in general have not caused difficulties in my patients. I recommend that they chew them well to play it safe or avoid them entirely if they are too anxious about eating them.

A high-fat diet. A large prospective study showed a direct relationship between fat intake, particularly red meat, and symptomatic diverticular disease.

HIGH-FIBER MENU PLAN

For those of you who have diverticular disease, I did not remove all foods with seeds from the menu plan. Personally, I haven't found them to be a problem, but if your doctor has advised you to avoid them or you simply feel safer not eating items with seeds, then certainly swap out the item for something else high in fiber.

Day 1

Breakfast (425)
1 cup bran cereal flakes (190)
1 cup skim milk (90)
3 large fresh figs (60)
½ cup orange juice with pulp (60)
1 teaspoon honey (25)
1 cup green tea

Lunch (463)
1 serving *Healthy Turkey Salad Pocket* (233) (page 335)
1 serving *Bean-Corn Salad* (120) (page 290)
5 dried plums (110)
1½ cups water with lemon

Midday Snack (320)
1 serving *Blackberry Smoothie* (320) (page 258)

Dinner (572)
1 serving *Winter White Bean Chili* (257) (page 282)
2 cups spinach salad with assorted veggies and 1 serving *Sweet Vidalia Onion Slaw with Fennel, Cucumber, and Champagne-Orange Dressing* (page 297) topped with 1 tablespoon ground flaxseeds (315)
1½ cups water with lemon

Evening Snack (230)
½ cup carrot sticks (50)
2 tablespoons hummus (50)
1 serving *Apple-Soy Chai Latte* (130) (page 254)

Day 2

Breakfast (600)
1 serving *Soufflé Omelet with Balsamic Strawberries* (160)
(page 345)
1 serving *Nutty Good Millet Muffins* (240) (page 352)
5 dried plums (110)
1 cup skim milk (90)

Lunch (390)
1 *Strawberry-Papaya Smoothie* (130) (page 255)
1 serving *Avocado-Fennel Citrus Salad* (page 285) topped with
½ cup kidney beans (225)
1 Wasa fiber crispbread (35)
1½ cups iced tea

Midday Snack (290)
1 serving *Rosemary Nuts* (290) (page 269)
1 cup green tea

Dinner (574)
1 serving *Cocoa-Encrusted Salmon with Blueberries* (270)
(page 330)
1 serving *Roasted Autumn Vegetables in Sherry Sauce* (114)
(page 360)
1 whole grain roll (100)
1 cup skim milk (90)

Evening Snack (240)
1 serving *Beanie-Greenie Brownies* (110) (page 309)
1 serving *Apple-Soy Chai Latte* (130) (page 254)

Day 3

Breakfast (498)
1 serving *Triple-Grain Georgia Pecan Pancakes* (188)
(page 346)
½ cup hash browns prepared with skins on (120)
1 cup Concord grapes (100)
1 cup skim milk (90)

Lunch (556)
1 serving *Asian Satay Skewers with Black Bean Sauce* (196)
(page 263)
1 serving *Raw Kale Salad with Lemon-Honey Vinaigrette* (260)
(page 296)
1 whole grain roll (100)
1½ cups water with lemon

Midday Snack (140)
1 serving *Winter Squash Soup with Roasted Seeds* (70)
(page 277)
1 serving *Cheese-and-Fruit Kebabs* (70) (page 272)
1½ cups water with lemon

Dinner (510)
1 serving *Chicken Thighs with Red Wine, Dried Plums, and
Garlic* (310) (page 323)
1 serving *Sicilian Broccoli Salad* (200) (page 291)
1 cup decaffeinated green tea

Evening Snack (290)
1 serving *Powerhouse Dried Plum Bars* (200) (page 343)
1 cup skim milk (90)

Leslie Bonci's Top Ten Tips for Constipation

Leslie Bonci, MPH, RD, is the director of Sports Medicine Nutrition at the University of Pittsburgh Medical Center and the author of the American Dietetic Association Guide to Better Digestion.

1. *Move it!* Don't forget that your gut is a muscle and if you sit all day, not only are you sluggish, but so is your digestive tract, so off the couch, out the door. Studies suggest that sedentary people are three times more likely to report constipation, and the lack of exercise is associated with a greater risk of forming diverticula.

2. *Get adequate rest!*

3. *Stop, drop, and go!* The longer you delay going to the toilet once you feel the urge, the more water that's absorbed from stool and the harder it becomes. Additionally, people who ignore the urge to have a bowel movement may eventually stop feeling the need to have one.

4. *Drink up.* Try to have liquid with every meal and snack, and incorporate some liquid foods, such as soups and chili, into your diet, in addition to water, skim milk, and vegetable juices. Hot tea or coffee can increase gastric motility.

5. *Include foods with fiber at every meal,* but if you don't eat a lot of fiber now, add it in *slowly*. Maybe 3- to 5-gram increments per week. So, if you currently consume 5 grams of fiber a day, increase to 8, and then to 11, 14, etc., until you get up to the recommended amount, which is 25 to 28 grams for men and 21 to 25 grams for women. But don't put all your bran in one bowl! Think oatmeal with a sprinkle of bran, or barley instead of rice, or add beans to a salad or soup. And eat the skins of potatoes or the peel of an apple.

6. *Dried plums.* Yes, formerly known as prunes, these little treasures can help with laxation. They are sweet, chewy, and a nat-

ural source of sorbitol. No need to eat a lot of them. Three to four should work fine. If you like, prune juice can be used as an alternative.

7. *Ground flaxseeds.* Start with one tablespoon and work your way up to two tablespoons added to hot cereal, a smoothie, soup, or stew.

8. *Black licorice.* I'm not talking Twizzlers here, but real black licorice; a few pieces may help to move things along.

9. *Make sure your diet is not* too low *in fat.* Fat can act as a lubricant, so a little olive oil, nuts, seeds, or nut butter can help with constipation.

10. Do a food swap to increase fiber at every meal:

- Barley for white rice
- Whole wheat bread instead of white
- Lentil soup instead of vegetable soup
- Bean dip for whole grain chips instead of a sour cream dip

DIARRHEA

Hey, "It" Happens

Did you know . . . the average adult has a bout of acute diarrhea at least four times a year? Close to 100 million cases of infectious diarrhea happen each year, resulting in over 3,000 deaths in the United States alone.

Optimal Food/Nutrient Highlights

Barley, rice, apples, tea, toast, carob, chocolate, probiotics and prebotics, yogurt.

What Is Diarrhea?

Diarrhea is an episode of loose, frequent, and watery stools that can happen infrequently or even daily. Acute diarrhea can last up to several days; diarrhea that lasts several weeks is labeled as chronic and is usually associated with more serious underlying health concerns.

An individual who has diarrhea typically passes stool more than three times a day. In more severe cases, they may pass more than a quart of stool in a day. Dehydration and lowered sodium and potassium levels are often the most critical situations that happen with diarrhea. Chronic diarrhea can also result in malnutrition, diminished appetite, and poor nutrient absorption in the digestive tract.

Common tests for determining the cause of diarrhea are

Stool culture. The laboratory checks for the presence of bacteria, parasites, or other signs of disease and infection.

Blood tests examine if there may be an underlying infection— white blood cell counts may be elevated.

Fasting tests can determine if a food intolerance or allergy is causing the diarrhea.

Sigmoidoscopy or colonoscopy. The doctor uses a special instrument that takes a video of the inside of the colon, which allows him to see the extent and location of damage.

Diagnostic imaging tests can determine if there are abnormal growths present.

What Causes It?

In most cases of acute diarrhea, there is an infection present that can be bacterial, viral, or parasitic in nature. The cause can often be traced back to poor hygiene, unclean conditions, or consumption of tainted foods or beverages. Chronic diarrhea is generally caused by a digestive disorder such as irritable bowel syndrome or by inflammatory bowel diseases such as colitis and Crohn's disease.

Another type of diarrhea, called osmotic diarrhea, is usually caused by eating foods or drinking beverages that contain substances that are not completely broken down. This has an often immediate laxative effect in the bowel. A category of sweeteners called sugar alcohols (examples include maltitol, sorbitol, and xylitol, found in gum and candies) often causes diarrhea when consumed by those who have difficulties digesting these sweeteners. Those who have lactose (the type of sugar found in milk) intolerance are either missing or not producing enough of the enzyme lactase, which is responsible for breaking down the sugar into a digestible form the body can handle. When the offending food or substance is removed from the diet, the diarrhea often stops.

Secretory diarrhea happens when excess fluid is drawn into the bowel by a variety of factors, such as medication side effects, inflammatory bowel diseases such as Crohn's and celiac, undigested fats, and wasting diseases such as AIDS and cancer.

Optimal Life Foods

For acute diarrhea, your doctor may advise you to give the bowel a rest by avoiding food entirely and suggest drinking lots of fluids. When it is time to introduce food again, probably the most popular diet for combating diarrhea is the BRAT diet. The acronym represents several of the 101 foods: **B**ananas, **R**ice (either white or brown), **A**pples (in the form of applesauce), **T**ea and/or **T**oast. (The toast should be white, not whole wheat.... I know, I know, but this is the only place you will see a recommendation for white bread, because it works!) When normal bowel movements resume, slowly introduce solid foods as tolerated, with an emphasis on keeping fat, fiber, and lactose-containing dairy products to a minimum.

Here are some other foods that I have found to be very helpful in dealing with diarrhea:

Probiotic foods like yogurt, kefir, and unpasteurized miso. Carob, chocolate (cocoa nibs work great and they are not loaded with lots of extra fat and sugar), honey, agave, bananas, and soy are prebiotic foods that help friendly bacteria take hold in the bowel.

Optimal Life Supplements

Psyllium. Although often used to promote bowel movements, this bulking agent has also been shown to help absorb excess fluid and add consistency to stools.

Saccharomyces boulardii. This yeast strain has been used successfully in treating diarrhea, especially that associated with *Clostridium difficile* infections, by reducing stool frequency and duration.

Caution! *Avoid herbal laxatives and supplements containing lactose, fructose, sugar alcohols, or caffeine or other stimulants.*

Feeding the Fire!

The following are best to avoid when experiencing diarrhea:

Liquids and other foods high in simple carbohydrates (lactose, sucrose, fructose) and sugar alcohols (sorbitol, xylitol, mannitol).

Caffeine-containing products.

Alcoholic beverages.

High-fiber and gas-producing foods such as nuts, beans, corn, broccoli, cauliflower, and cabbage. Foods that contain less than two grams of fiber per serving are ideal.

Raw fruits and vegetables, with the exception of bananas, melons, and lettuce.

Fried foods.

Spicy foods if not tolerated.

Any foods that you think may be making matters worse—when in doubt, leave it out!

ANTIDIARRHEAL MENU PLAN

Day 1

Breakfast (382)
1½ cups puffed rice (82)
1 cup rice milk (130)
½ cup low-sugar fruit cocktail (70)
½ cup pear nectar (75)
1 teaspoon honey (25)
1 cup green tea

Lunch (415)
1 cup chicken noodle soup (120)
½ ounce pretzels (55)
4 ounces high-probiotic fruited yogurt (110)
1 cup carob rice milk (130)

Midday Snack (220)
½ cup applesauce (90)
1 cup carob rice milk (130)

Dinner (450)
1 cup miso soup (35)
4 ounces rotisserie chicken (220)
½ cup steamed green beans (25)
½ cup brown rice (100)
½ cup Concord grape juice (70)

Evening Snack (480)
1 cup kefir (210)
5 gingersnap cookies (140)
1 cup carob rice milk (130)

Day 2

Breakfast (530)
2 scrambled eggs (omega-3 enriched) with 1 slice rice cheese (210)
½ banana (60)
1 slice toast with 1 teaspoon grape jelly (105)
1 cup carob rice milk (130)
1 teaspoon honey (25)
1 cup green tea

Lunch (500)
1 cup chicken rice soup (110)
½ turkey sandwich on white bread (190)
½ cup low-sugar canned peaches (70)
1 cup carob rice milk (130)

Midday Snack (241)
1 ounce cocoa nibs (171)
½ cup low-sugar fruit cocktail (70)

Dinner (500)
1 serving *Irish Poached Salmon* (350) (page 320)
1 white dinner roll (100)
½ cup cooked carrot coins and green beans (25)
1 teaspoon honey (25)
1 cup decaffeinated green tea

Evening Snack (240)
4 ounces high-probiotic fruited yogurt (110)
1 cup carob rice milk (130)

_____

Day 3

Breakfast (515)
2 (4-inch) wheat pancakes (170)
1 slice whole grain toast (80)
1 scrambled egg (omega-3 enriched) (75)
½ banana (60)
1 cup carob rice milk (130)

Lunch (336)
1 cup miso soup with ¼ cup cubed firm tofu (79)
8 tamari rice crackers (56)
½ cup Asian-blend cooked vegetables (25)
½ cup applesauce (90)
1 cup carob rice milk (130)

Midday Snack (220)
1 serving *Apple-Soy Chai Latte* (130) (page 254)
½ cup applesauce (90)

Dinner (695)
1 serving *Cocoa-Encrusted Salmon with Blueberries* (270)
(page 330)
½ cup brown rice (100)
½ cup steamed carrots (25)
½ cup applesauce (90)
1 slice whole wheat toast (80)
1 cup carob rice milk (130)
1 cup water

Evening Snack (210)
3 cups air-popped popcorn with butter spray (80)
1 serving *Apple-Soy Chai Latte* (130) (page 254)

Dave's Tips

1. Eat small, frequent meals and snacks every three or four hours
   and drink plenty of fluids.
2. Avoid oils and fats until your stool is formed.
3. Avoid sugary high-fructose drinks, candy, and alcohol.
4. No raw fruits and vegetables, except bananas.

GASTROESOPHAGEAL REFLUX DISEASE (GERD)

Burn, Baby, Burn

Did you know... 45 percent of all Americans experience heartburn at least once per month and more children than ever before are being diagnosed with acid reflux disease?

Optimal Food/Nutrient Highlights

Low-glycemic, high-fiber, and pectin-rich foods, fatty fish, blackberries, carrots, kale, strawberries, teff, apples, cranberries, cardamom, magnesium, melatonin.

What Is Gastroesophageal Reflux Disease?

Reflux (aka "heartburn") happens when a muscle called the lower esophageal sphincter (LES), whose purpose is to keep the contents of the stomach in the stomach, fails to work. Then, acidy contents flow back up into the esophagus, causing the inside lining to experience the classic "burn." Although everyone experiences an occasional bout of reflux, if it occurs often, severe damage can happen to the lining of the esophagus from acid erosion. If there are more than two occurrences of reflux a week, it is called gastroesophageal reflux disease (GERD). When the lining of the esophagus starts to bleed or ulcers form, this is known as esophagitis.

Untreated, constant damage to the esophagus creates scar tissue, causing the passageway to narrow and requiring medical intervention to dilate the esophagus. If this vicious cycle is not broken, cells that line the inside of the esophagus become further damaged and subject to mutation, which can lead to a pre-cancerous condition called Barrett's esophagus. Once diagnosed, those who have Barrett's esophagus are thirty to seventy-five times more likely to develop esophageal cancer than those who do not have it.

Reflux can also bring about other health conditions and symptoms, including asthma, persistent sore throat, hoarseness, chronic cough, chest pain, feeling of a lump in the throat, sensation of food coming back into the mouth, and an acid or bitter taste in the mouth. Symptoms of reflux can last for minutes, hours, or days and are usually more pronounced at night, especially after lying down after a large meal.

What Causes It?

There are several contributing factors to why people develop reflux disease; however, rising obesity seems to explain rising rates of reflux and GERD. Members of the same family may also be diagnosed with it, so there may be genetic factors involved. Other contributing factors include hiatal hernia, pregnancy, smoking, diabetes, and delayed stomach emptying (which may be a side effect of some medications).

Optimal Life Foods

Low-glycemic foods (whole grains, most fruit and vegtables).

High-fiber and pectin-rich foods (whole grains, guavas, papaya, dried plums, flaxseed, beans, passion fruit, persimmons).

Foods high in omega-3 (omega-3 eggs, flaxseed, fatty fish).

Blackberries help heal the esophagus and may decrease risk of esophageal cancer.

Carrots, kale, strawberries, and teff may reduce risk of esophageal cancer.

Apples, cranberries, and cardamom help combat heartburn and gastritis.

Optimal Life Supplements

Melatonin may protect against damage to the lining of the esophagus by reducing inflammatory prostaglandins.

Magnesium. This mineral is essential for relaxation of smooth muscles, including the large intestine, and it also can have a slight laxative effect.

Deglycyrrhizinated licorice, or DGL, can soothe indigestion by increasing the mucous lining.

Slippery elm. This herbal remedy comes from the inner bark of the red elm tree. It is soothing and protective for mucosal tissue.

Chamomile is one of the most calming herbs for the stomach.

Selenium helps fight esophageal cancer.

Digestive enzymes break down carbohydrates, protein, and fat and help move food through the digestive system. These are essential ingredients to protect and aid in the repair of the lining of the esophagus.

A *multivitamin* (iron-free), including buffered vitamin C, folate, vitamin B_6, beta-carotene, and selenium.

Omega-3 fish oil reduces inflammation.

Whey protein may help promote weight loss by encouraging lean muscle tissue to grow.

Psyllium fiber promotes good digestion.

Rice bran works like a sponge and absorbs excess acid in the stomach.

Kudzu root also does a great job in reducing stomach acid.

Caution! *Dietary supplements that contain caffeine such as ephedra, bissy nut, and guarana, and also mint-flavored supplements, can contribute to reflux.*

Feeding the Fire!

The following foods may contribute to symptoms of GERD. However, my experience has been that these foods are not problematic for everyone. Try eliminating them either all at once or one at a time, depending on how patient you are with your discomfort.

Black and red pepper.

Caffeinated beverages (regular tea, coffee, colas, energy drinks).

Decaffeinated coffee and tea beverages can trigger GERD symptoms. Try herbal teas instead, except those containing peppermint or spearmint.

Alcohol is one of the worst things to consume if you have GERD.

Chocolate can also spur on reflux, but like most things that are decadent, it may be a matter of portion size. Try less than an ounce a day if you can't live without chocolate, and if it doesn't bother you, enjoy!

Mint such as peppermint and spearmint lowers LES pressure and allows acid to splash back into the esophagus.

High-fat foods slow down the emptying of contents of the stomach, placing more pressure on the LES.

Tomatoes, citrus, garlic, onions, spicy foods, and condiments such as ketchup, mustard, and vinegar often aggravate GERD.

Carbonated beverages create more gas and distension in the stomach.

ANTI-GERD MENU PLAN

Day 1

Breakfast (435)
1 cup flaxseed cereal flakes with dried cranberries (250)
1 cup skim milk (90)
½ cup Concord grape juice (70)
1 teaspoon honey (25)
1 cup chamomile tea

Lunch (353)
1 serving *Healthy Turkey Salad Pocket* (233) (page 335)
1 serving *Slow-Cooker Sweet Potatoes* (70) (page 368)
1 cup strawberries (50)
1½ cups water

Midday Snack (320)
1 serving *Blackberry Smoothie* (page 258), substituting
½ medium banana for the orange juice (320)

Dinner (550)
4 ounces rotisserie chicken (220)
1 serving *Curried Chickpeas and Kale* (150) (page 370)
1 cup steamed Brussels sprouts (60)
½ cup corn polenta (120)
1½ cups water

Evening Snack (370)
1 serving *Nutty Good Millet Muffins* (240) (page 352)
1 serving *Apple-Soy Chai Latte* (130) (page 254)

Day 2

Breakfast (510)
2 scrambled omega-3 eggs (150)
1 whole wheat English muffin with jelly (135)
5 dried plums (110)
1 cup skim milk (90)
1 teaspoon honey (25)
1 cup chamomile tea

Lunch (450)
1 serving *Sweet Vidalia Onion Slaw with Fennel, Cucumber, and Champagne-Orange Dressing* (250) (page 297)
1 serving *Winter Squash Soup with Roasted Seeds* (70) (page 277)
1 serving *Cheese-and-Fruit Kebabs* (70) (page 272)
½ cup papaya juice (60)
1½ cups water

Midday Snack (140)
1 serving *Christine's Baked Custard* (140) (page 308)

Dinner (730)
1 serving *Irish Poached Salmon* (page 320) with *Yogurt Sauce* (page 305) (380)
1 serving *Barley Salad with Edamame* (160) (page 287)
1 whole grain roll (100)
1 cup skim milk (90)

Evening Snack (110)
1 serving *Beanie-Greenie Brownies* (110) (page 309)
1 cup chamomile tea

Day 3

Breakfast (410)
1 serving *Creamy Cherry Oatmeal* (210) (page 350)
1 cup diced mango (110)
1 cup skim milk (90)
1 cup chamomile tea

Lunch (623)
1 serving *Healthy Turkey Salad Pocket* (233) (page 335)
1 serving *Summer Fruits Pie* (390) (page 315)
1½ cups water

Midday Snack (130)
1 serving *Strawberry-Papaya Smoothie* (130) (page 255)

Dinner (650)
1 serving *Asparagus-Sesame Stir-Fry* (100) (page 362); for more
protein, add 4 ounces tuna, tempeh, or tofu to the recipe (100)
½ cup brown rice (100)
1 serving *Nuts and Berry Fruit Salad* (350) (page 286)
1½ cups water

Evening Snack (230)
1 serving *Quick Pumkin Smoothie* (230) (page 256)

Dave's Tips

1. Losing weight (if overweight) has a significant impact on GERD.
   The incidence of GERD has risen with obesity rates.
2. Eat small, frequent meals (five to six per day). Big meals, especially late at night before bedtime, cause gastric distention and

allow the lower esophageal sphincter to relax, which lets acid back into the esophagus. Remain upright after eating. Avoid lying down for three hours after a meal.

3. Stopping smoking decreases pressure on the sphincter that contributes to reflux.
4. Get in seven to eight hours of sleep and raise the head of your bed six to eight inches by putting blocks of wood under the bedposts. Sleeping on your left side also helps reduce LES pressure.
5. Keep a food journal to pinpoint offending foods.

HALITOSIS (BAD BREATH)

Scared to Breath(e)?

Did you know... almost everyone at one time or another experiences *halitophobia* ("fear of having bad breath")? It is estimated that about 25 percent of the population has experienced chronic bad breath at some time, yet most people are unable to tell if they have it, even if they do.

Optimal Food/Nutrient Highlights

Water, gum, mint, cinnamon, guavas, ginger, basil, green tea, wasabi, cranberries, cherries, yogurt, honey, agave, cardamom, digestive enzymes, probiotics, vitamin C, bioflavonoids, CoQ_{10}, fiber.

What Is Halitosis?

Halitosis is the medical word for "bad breath." *Halitosis* is derived from the Latin word *halitus*, which means "breath," and the Greek suffix *osis,* which means "condition." I'm not talking the occasional morning breath or the kind of breath you get after eating a meal loaded with garlic and onions. In fact, more than *90 million* people suffer from chronic halitosis and the numbers have been increasing in the past few decades. By the way, *you* are not the best judge of whether you have it or not, as you may have become accustomed to the odor. Loved ones, and certainly your doctor, are better judges.

What Causes It?

In the majority of cases, bad breath originates from the gums and tongue, where decaying food particles or other substances in the mouth form anaerobic bacteria. These bacteria produce sulfur compounds as a by-product of the proteins as they decay.

The major causes of halitosis include poor oral hygiene or poorly fitting dentures, gum disease, diabetes, kidney failure, liver disease, xerostomia (dry mouth due to insufficent saliva), snoring, smoking, postnasal drip, stomach reflux or constipation (more rare), hunger/dieting/fasting, and side effects from medications.

Optimal Life Foods

Water. Drink plenty of fluids, including water! Keeping well hydrated helps reduce "empty stomach" breath.

Gum. I know what you're thinking. It's not really a "food," but chewing gum has been found to keep the mouth moist and reduce bacteria, especially the cinnamon variety. A study by researchers at the University of Illinois found that a popular cinnamon-flavored chewing gum reduced bad-breath-causing bacteria in the back of the mouth by 43 percent!

Mint helps freshen breath while killing underlying bacteria that cause odor. It also aids in digestion.

Cinnamon. This spice contains cinnamic aldehyde, a plant essential oil that kills bacteria.

Guavas, ginger, basil, green tea, and wasabi (a Japanese condiment similar to horseradish) were found, in a study, to inhibit bacteria that form oral plaque.

Cranberries and cherries make plaque-promoting bacteria "less sticky," therefore less likely to accumulate in the mouth.

Yogurt. I recommend eating at least six ounces of a low-sugar yogurt to all of my patients challenged with bad breath. One of the offending smells associated with bad breath is hydrogen sulfide. Japanese researchers found that yogurt reduces hydrogen sulfide by over 80 percent and also reduces the gingivitis and plaque that often accompany bad breath.

Honey and agave are two of my favorite sweeteners because they are delicious and also have antibacterial properties.

Cardamom contains cineole, which has antiseptic properties just like mouthwash.

Parsley and fennel have traditionally been used in various cultures to help fight bad breath. However, research has found these are ineffective in fighting odor-causing bacteria, but may merely provide temporary relief.

Optimal Life Supplements

Digestive enzymes plus probiotics are highly recommended if GERD/digestive disorders are suspected.

Vitamin C, bioflavonoids, and CoQ$_{10}$ do a great job in protecting gums from disease and also in repairing gums that are diseased.

Fiber fights chronic constipation, which can be a contributor to bad breath.

Caution! *Chewable dietary supplements with high sugar content can feed bacteria. There are odorless versions of garlic supplements, but instead of smelling it on your breath, others may detect the distinct odor coming through your skin!*

Feeding the Fire!

Coffee, black tea, spicy foods (including onions and garlic), sugary foods (bacteria feed on sugar), *and alcohol and high-protein, low-carb diets* (these cause ketosis, a process of rapid fat breakdown) exacerbate halitosis.

SWEET BREATH MENU PLAN

Day 1

Breakfast (355)
1 cup flaxseed cereal flakes (190)
1 cup skim milk (90)
1 kiwi (50)
1 teaspoon honey (25)
1 cup green tea

Lunch (505)
1 serving *Christine's Yummy Bean and Cheese Tostada* (260)
(page 319)

½ ounce whole grain pretzels (55)
1 cup strawberries (50)
1 serving *Christine's Baked Custard* (140) (page 308)
1 cup green tea with lemon

Midday Snack (220)
1 serving *Chilean Fruit Guacamole* (100) (page 259)
12 fat-free corn chips (120)
1½ cups sparkling water with lime

Dinner (520)
4 ounces rotisserie chicken (220)
1 cup steamed Brussels sprouts (60)
½ cup corn polenta (120)
2 cups spinach salad with assorted veggies and citrus dressing (120)

Evening Snack (370)
1 sliced apple and 2 tablespoons almond butter sprinkled with cinnamon (260)
4 ounces high-probiotic yogurt (110)
1 cup decaffeinated green tea

Day 2

Breakfast (495)
1 serving *Soufflé Omelet with Balsamic Strawberries* (160) (page 345)
1 slice whole grain toast with 1 teaspoon mint jelly (105)
5 dried plums (100)
1 serving *Apple-Soy Chai Latte* (130) (page 254)

Lunch (400)

5 ounces California-roll sushi with wasabi (300)

1 cup miso soup (100)

1 cup green tea

Midday Snack (290)

1 serving *Rosemary Nuts* (290) (page 269)

1 cup green tea

Dinner (670)

1 serving *Cocoa-Encrusted Salmon with Blueberries* (270)
(page 330)

1 serving *Asparagus-Carrot Rolls* (210) (page 361)

1 whole grain roll (100)

1 cup skim milk (90)

1 cup decaffeinated green tea

Evening Snack (110)

1 serving *Beanie-Greenie Brownies* (110) (page 309)

1 cup decaffeinated green tea

Day 3

Breakfast (490)

Yogurt, fresh cherries, and 1 serving *Cherry–Chai Spice
Granola* (page 348) (make a parfait out of the three!) (400)

1 slice whole wheat toast (60)

1 serving *Fruit and Walnut Jam Conserve* (30) (page 302)

1 cup green tea

Lunch (430)

1 serving *Winter Squash Soup with Roasted Seeds* (70) (page 277)

1 serving *Raw Kale Salad with Lemon-Honey Vinaigrette* (260)
(page 296)
1 whole grain roll (100)
1 cup green tea

Midday Snack (192)
1 serving *Cherry Zinger Smoothie* (192) (page 256)

Dinner (656)
1 serving *Dilled Salmon Cakes* (180) (page 328)
1 serving *Quinoa Pilaf with Currants and Turmeric* (320)
(page 369)
1 serving *Avocado-Fennel Citrus Salad* (120) (page 285)
1 serving *Watermelon Soda* (36) (page 253)

Evening Snack (130)
1 serving *Spicy Biscotti* (130) (page 311)
1 cup decaffeinated green tea

Dave's Tips

1. Eat small, frequent meals because an empty stomach can contribute to odor.
2. Choose more plant-based proteins, which are rich in fiber, to aid digestive health.
3. Use agave, honey, or noncaloric sweeteners to reduce the fuel (sugar) that bacteria feed on.
4. Drink lots of water between meals to avoid dry mouth syndrome.
5. Chew cinnamon gum between meals!

GAS

"Better to Have an Empty House Than an Angry Tenant!"

Did you know... most people pass gas around ten times a day, regardless of age or gender? But even up to twenty times a day would be considered "normal." The volume of gas released per person per day often ranges anywhere from a cup to as much as one-half gallon.

Optimal Food/Nutrient Highlights

Rice, peppermint, fennel, yogurt, kefir, ginger, probiotics, digestive enzymes.

What Is Gas?

"Gas," or flatus, is formed in the stomach or intestine and is made up of (usually) odorless vapors such as carbon dioxide, oxygen, nitrogen, hydrogen, and sometimes methane. Flatulence is gas passed through the anus. Expelling these vapors from the stomach through the mouth is referred to as belching.

Gas can be problematic for those who have physical pain and discomfort when gas is withheld and becomes trapped, causing pressure and pain in the bowel.

What Causes It?

Gas generally occurs because

You swallowed air while eating or you consumed carbonated beverages.

You ate indigestible carbohydrates. Because the human body cannot digest and absorb some carbohydrates (because we lack the enzymes to break them down in the small intestine), they go "undigested" into the large intestine, where friendly bacteria help to break down these carbohydrates by fermenting them. This creates mostly hydrogen, carbon dioxide, and methane gases.

Following are the carbohydrates behind all of the rumblings:

- *Raffinose* describes a family of oligosaccharides, or natural sugars, found in beans, mushrooms, and various other vegetables and grains. Other animals have an enzyme called alpha-galactosidase to digest these carbohydrates, but unfortunately, we do not.
- *Fructose,* though naturally present in a variety of foods, including fruits, is found in much higher percentages in some foods than in others. High-fructose foods include artichokes, asparagus, leeks, onions, pears, watermelon, apples, honeydew, dried fruits, and wheat. Although, ironically, high-fructose corn syrup sweetener may actually contain less fructose than the aforementioned foods, it is still a source of fructose and may contribute to gas.
- *Lactose* is a natural sugar found in a variety of dairy products, such as milk, cheese, and ice cream. Certain segments of the population, particularly those of African, Asian, and southern European descent, do not produce or produce insufficient levels of the lactase enzyme that breaks down lactose.
- *Sorbitol,* considered a sugar alcohol, is found naturally in a variety of fruits, including apples, pears, peaches, and dried plums (prunes). Sorbitol is often used as an artificial sweetener and can cause flatulence at varying levels of intake depending on the individual. Other sugar alcohols may cause gas too.

You ate foods high in fiber. Many foods that are considered "healthy," including vegetables, fruits, whole grains, and beans, are high in fiber and may be the biggest contributors to gas. However, gas may occur because of a sudden introduction of fiber, to which your body hasn't had time to adjust. One study found that daily consumption of one-half cup of pinto beans or vegetarian baked beans increased flatulence among participants. However, flatulence diminished by the second to fourth weeks of consumption.

You are taking a medication that causes gas.

You have a medical condition that causes gas. Celiac disease, irritable bowel syndrome (IBS), GERD, and many other conditions of the digestive system can cause gas.

Optimal Life Foods

Rice is one of the few grains known not to cause gas. Rice flour works like a sponge to absorb gas.

Peppermint has been shown to improve IBS symptoms such as gas.

Fennel tea has been used for centuries to help relieve indigestion.

Yogurt and kefir are cultured dairy products that are abundantly available and are easy and delicious ways of introducing helpful bacteria that reduce gas.

Ginger is a wonderful aid to digestion.

Optimal Life Supplements

Probiotics is another term for "friendly bacteria," which help maintain a healthy lower bowel by keeping harmful bacteria at bay. Research has shown that probiotics can help reduce flatulence and bloating.

Digestive enzymes. A broad-spectrum digestive enzyme that aids in the breakdown of carbohydrates, protein, and fat can be helpful.

Slippery elm is an herb aptly named for its "slippery" feel when it is chewed or mixed with water. It is useful for treating a variety of inflammatory digestive disorders.

Beano is a product containing the enzyme alpha-galactosidase, which is derived from the fungus *Aspergillus niger.* Alpha-galactosidase helps break down indigestible oligosaccharides.

Caution! *Garlic, fish oil, multivitamins, psyllium husk fiber, and some herbal preparations may cause gas. Activated charcoal is effective orally for combating gas, but it can interfere with so many medications and dietary supplements that it may not be worth it.*

Feeding the Fire!

These foods may cause flatulence in some people, but may not produce flatulence in others.

Beans.

Dairy (if lactose intolerant) such as milk, ice cream, and cheese.

Vegetables. Gassy varieties include garlic, onions, leeks, cabbage, broccoli, celery, radishes, Brussels sprouts, cauliflower, kale, cucumbers, sauerkraut, eggplant, artichokes, and asparagus.

Fruits such as melons, apricots, apples, and pears, as well as raisins, dried plums, and other dried fruits, can contribute to gas.

Whole grains such as wheat, wheat products, and bran.

Nuts and seeds.

Carbonated beverages such as soda, beer, and carbonated water.

Bonnie Taub-Dix's Top Ten Tips for Gas and Bloating

Bonnie Taub-Dix, MA, RD, is a national spokesperson for the American Dietetic Association and coauthor of Kosher by Design Lightens Up: Fabulous Food for a Healthier Lifestyle.

1. *Eat with your mouth closed.* Drinking through a straw or from the mouth of a bottle or a water fountain, chewing gum, and eating with your mouth open introduce air into the stomach. Loose-fitting dentures and cigarette smoking can also entrap air.

2. *Slow down!* Although air is swallowed whenever a person eats or drinks, gulping food and eating too quickly will cause more air to be swallowed. Eat more slowly and try to enjoy each bite without rushing through your meal. It's also important to eat smaller meals more frequently—don't skip meals or go for long periods of time without eating. Eating in an unbalanced fashion may not only trap air, but also trap unwanted extra pounds, since slower eaters are usually slimmer.

3. *Tea tames tummy troubles.* Teas like chamomile, anise, ginger, and peppermint are soothing, and a steamy mug can help cut gas and bloat. If you suffer from gastro-esophageal reflux disease (GERD), however, avoid peppermint-containing foods.

4. *Bubbles bloat.* Try avoiding carbonated beverages, which can fill you with gas (carbon dioxide). Be aware of foods that have air incorporated into them such as whipped cream, soft-serve frozen yogurt, milkshakes, and malteds.

5. *One at a time.* There's good news and bad news about gassy foods: The bad news is that they can make you feel bloated and uncomfortable, but the good news is that they're so good for you! Try not to consume more than one food known to cause

gas at a time so your body can become adjusted to it. Watch your fat intake, too, since fatty foods move slowly through the digestive tract, allowing more time for fermentation and gas production.

6. *"Dairy" good approach.* Just because lactose found in milk and milk products can cause gas, there's no need to avoid these calcium-rich foods. Over-the-counter enzymes that help digest lactose are readily available, as are a host of other lactose-free food products.

7. *Move it to lose it.* Exercise is a great way to stimulate the passage of gas through the digestive tract. Physical activity can also relieve anxiety and reduce stress-induced abdominal pain, since people tend to swallow more air when they're nervous. Avoid tight-fitting garments, girdles, and belts and try not to lie down right after eating.

8. *Stay the course.* Fiber can create abdominal distention, particularly when you're consuming soluble fiber (oat bran, beans, peas) versus insoluble fiber (wheat bran). A slow introduction of fiber-rich foods, gradually working yourself up to twenty-five to thirty-five grams per day, can help ease digestion and minimize gas. Always be sure to drink plenty of fluids when increasing your fiber intake.

9. *Talk to an expert.* Certain medications can interrupt the normal process of digestion, including common antibiotics. Antacids aid in calming a gassy stomach by breaking up bubbles, and probiotics may soothe your symptoms by providing "friendly bacteria" for your system. It's best to check with your physician or a registered dietitian before taking over-the-counter medications.

10. *Track it down.* Keeping a daily food diary can be incredibly helpful in tracking the foods you eat and identifying the symptoms they create. Use a simple key next to each meal (e.g., G =

gas, B = bloat, P = pain) to help you focus in on your individual food intolerances and eating styles. Be sure to also note the timing of your meals, the quantities of food consumed, and where the meals were eaten (in a relaxing restaurant, at your desk, or standing in front of the refrigerator). Although some people feel that a food journal is a pain to maintain, it could help save you a lot of the other "pain" in the long run.

LESS GASSY MENU PLAN

This menu is most certainly a high-fiber plan, but if you take a slow-but-sure approach and gradually ramp up your fiber intake, you should be less "windy." I also took the liberty of adding in two tablespoons of beans at dinnertime each day. I want you to gradually increase your bean intake to a goal of one-half cup daily. Also, don't forget that the goal here is to be less gassy, not gas-free.

Day 1

Breakfast (375)
1 cup flaxseed cereal flakes (190)
1 cup light soy milk (110)
1 cup strawberries (50)
1 teaspoon honey (25)
1 cup peppermint green tea

Lunch (535)
1 serving *Warm Goat Cheese Salad with Hazelnuts and Raspberries* (390) (page 295)

1 whole wheat roll (100)
½ cup sweet cherries (45)
1 cup iced ginger green tea

Midday Snack (296)
1 serving *Crumb-Topped Georgia Pecan and Cherry Cereal Bars* (216) (page 341)
1 cup skim milk (90)

Dinner (580)
4 ounces rotisserie chicken (220)
1 serving *Slow-Cooker Sweet Potatoes* (70) (page 367)
2 cups spinach salad with *Avocado Chimichurri* (page 300) sauce (120)
2 tablespoons beans of your choice (not green beans) (30)
1 serving *Christine's Baked Custard* (140) (page 308)
1 cup decaffeinated ginger green tea

Evening Snack (220)
1 serving *Chilean Fruit Guacamole* (100) (page 259)
12 fat-free corn chips (120)
1 cup decaffeinated peppermint green tea

Day 2

Breakfast (460)
1 serving *Soufflé Omelet with Balsamic Strawberries* (160) (page 345)
1 whole grain English muffin (100)
1 serving *Fruit and Walnut Jam Conserve* (30) (page 302)
1 cup diced papaya (60)
1 cup light soy milk (110)

Lunch (440)

1 serving *Blackberry Smoothie* (320) (page 258)

1 serving *Avocado-Fennel Citrus Salad* (120) (page 285)

Midday Snack (290)

1 serving *Rosemary Nuts* (290) (page 269)

1 cup peppermint green tea

Dinner (550)

1 serving *Dilled Salmon Cakes* (180) (page 328)

1 serving *Roasted Root Vegetables* (240) (page 365)

2 tablespoons beans of your choice (not green beans) (30)

1 whole grain roll (100)

1 cup decaffeinated ginger green tea

Evening Snack (240)

1 serving *Nutty Good Millet Muffins* (240) (page 352)

1 cup decaffeinated green tea

Day 3

Breakfast (358)

1 serving *Triple-Grain Georgia Pecan Pancakes* (188) (page 346)

1 orange (60)

1 cup light soy milk (110)

1 cup green tea

Lunch (535)

1 serving *Mango-Tango Tilapia Salad* (270) (page 288)

1 whole grain roll (100)

1 serving *Poached Pears* (165) (page 307)

1 cup peppermint green tea

Midday Snack (380)
1 serving *Chef Wiley's Granola* (290) (page 351)
1 cup skim milk (90)

Dinner (505)
1 serving *Grilled Chicken Salad with Pomegranate Vinaigrette and Mango Gelée Garnish* (300) (page 324)
2 tablespoons beans of your choice (not green beans) (30)
½ cup brown rice (100)
½ cup guava juice (75)

Evening Snack (260)
1 serving *Spicy Biscotti* (130) (page 311)
1 serving *Apple-Soy Chai Latte* (130) (page 254)

IRRITABLE BOWEL SYNDROME (IBS)

Look Out Below!

Did you know... irritable bowel syndrome (IBS), the most common diagnosed digestive disorder, affects nearly one out of ten people in the United States? Seventy percent of sufferers are women. About half of those with IBS are diagnosed before the age of thirty-five.

Optimal Food/Nutrient Highlights

Fiber, prebiotics, probiotics, kefir, peppermint, artichokes.

What Is Irritable Bowel Syndrome?

According to the National Institutes of Health, IBS refers to a complex disorder of the lower intestinal tract that is mainly characterized by a pattern of symptoms often worsened by emotional stress. Symptoms of IBS can include lower abdominal pain, constipation and/or diarrhea, bloating, mucus in the stools, excessive gas and gas pain, fatigue, and urinary incontinence.

In general, there are three basic categories of IBS:

- With constipation
- With diarrhea
- With both

IBS symptoms often vary from one person to another. For some, frequency and intensity of symptoms can vary with episodic periods of "remission," while others may experience a gradual worsening of symptoms over time. Though IBS is not considered to be life-threatening, those who have it would argue that their quality of life has been negatively impacted. Irritable bowel syndrome is often confused with more serious digestive disorders (collectively known as inflammatory bowel disease) such as Crohn's disease and ulcerative colitis.

A physician may prescribe tests including a stool sample, blood tests, X-rays, and colonoscopy and/or sigmoidoscopy to determine the cause of symptoms, but to date, there isn't one specific test for diagnosing IBS. Once a more serious digestive disorder is ruled out, the doctor may conclude you have IBS based on the list of symptoms above. In diarrheal IBS, it also makes sense to test for celiac disease.

What Causes It?

The precise cause of IBS is unknown, but there are several contributing factors under investigation. These include genetic predis-
position, increased levels of serotonin, elevated inflammatory
response to infection, increased sensitivity of the enteric nervous
system causing abnormal motility and pain, stress, anxiety, panic,
and depression.

In my experience, I have yet to meet a patient with IBS who did
not also present with the challenge of stress. We all exhibit the effects of stress in different ways. Some people get backaches or tension between the shoulder blades, some eat less, some eat more,
and those with IBS exhibit stress through their bowels. As you will
see further on, stress management is an integral tool in treating
IBS.

Optimal Life Foods

Because of the highly individualized nature of treating IBS, I
stongly recommend that you consult with a registered dietitian to
design an optimal program for you. In general, a minimum of three
visits after diagnosis with an RD is recommended to get you head-
ing down the right path. Besides an overall diet that is low in fat,
here are some foods that I have found helpful in controlling IBS.

Fiber. Though an overview of the literature that has examined the
effectiveness of fiber in treating IBS is somewhat mixed, the 2005
Dietary Guidelines for Americans recommends a level of twenty-five
to thirty-five grams per day. I have yet to meet a patient diagnosed
with IBS who was already meeting this recommended level of fiber,
as is true of most Americans! I suggest increasing fiber slowly to
the 25–35 g/day level as tolerated. For IBS with constipation, see

page 156 for a comprehensive list of high-fiber foods. For IBS with diarrhea, see page 166 for foods that benefit diarrhea.

Prebiotics and probiotics. Some research has found that foods containing prebiotics and probiotics provide relief of symptoms such as pain, gas, and stool frequency—more so with the bifidobacteria variety compared with lactobacillus-based probiotics. Though research is inconclusive at this point, I still feel that those foods rich in friendly bacteria can be a godsend for IBS sufferers. Examples include yogurt and kefir (both contain minimal if any lactose), sauerkraut, kimchi, and unpasteurized miso. There are also several fortified products on the market with a variety of different strains of potentially beneficial bacteria in them. Here is a list of some of the most beneficial strains of bacteria for digestive challenges:

- *Bifidobacterium animalis*
- *Bifidobacterium infantis*
- *Bifidobacterium lactis*
- *Lactobacillus casei*
- *Lactobacillus reuteri*
- *Saccharomyces boulardi* (considered a yeast, not a bacteria)

Peppermint oil was found to be more helpful in reducing symptoms of IBS when compared with a placebo.

Artichokes. Human studies have shown that artichoke-leaf extract may reduce the symptoms of IBS.

Optimal Life Supplements

Supplements to relieve constipation (see page 157).

Supplements to relieve diarrhea (see page 167).

Probiotics are naturally occurring in foods and are available in fortified foods and also as dietary supplements.

Artichoke-leaf extract. Ninety-six percent of patients surveyed in one study ranked artichoke-leaf extract as good as, if not better than, other medical options for treating IBS.

Caution! *Avoid supplements with excess caffeine, sorbitol, fructose, or lactose.*

Chinese herbal medicines. Some trials have shown effectiveness with their use, but due to the inconsistency of quality and availability, they are generally not recommended.

Feeding the Fire!

In the January 2009 issue of *The American Journal of Gastroenterology,* a review of eight studies that included 540 subjects concluded that there was a wide range of positive IBS symptom responses to "allergic foods" (anywhere from 12.5 percent to 67 percent). Because these studies lacked a control group, it is unknown if their response could be attributed to a placebo effect. My clinical experience has been that patients experience a variety of possible "food intolerances." Keeping a food diary to track nutritional intake along with matching symptoms would be the best approach to identifying specific foods that are problematic for you. Here are some possible offenders:

Beans, broccoli, Brussels sprouts, cabbage, cauliflower, corn, leeks, and onions are the most common offenders. These may need to be avoided only at the beginning of your new diet to "quiet the storm," but as you will see, gradually adding these foods back into the diet may be quite helpful in the overall management of IBS.

High-fat foods slow gastric emptying.

Carbonated beverages.

Fructose may produce gas.

Caffeine. High levels of caffeine can exert a laxative effect and for some can be constipating.

Alcohol irritates the lining of the digestive tract.

Lactose is generally a concern only if you are lactose intolerant.

Sorbitol is a common sugar alcohol found in sugar-free candies and gums. It can have a laxative effect on some, especially when consumed in quantity.

Raffinose is an indigestible carbohydrate found in beans.

Prune or grape juice can be more of a concern for IBS with diarrhea. White grape juice has a lower fructose content and may be better tolerated.

ANTI-IBS MENU PLAN

Since there are different types of IBS—with constipation, with diarrhea, or with both—refer to either the High-Fiber Menu Plan found on page 159 or the Antidiarrheal Menu Plan on page 168. If your IBS is the combo variety, begin with the Antidiarrheal Menu Plan, then slowly add in more high-fiber foods. The artichoke-leaf extract and probiotics really help in either scenario. And what makes this diet even more effective is eating in a calm, unhurried environment that is "stress-free." Stress and tension at the dinner table is an IBS sufferer's worst nightmare!

URINARY TRACT INFECTIONS (UTIs)

Fighting the Urge

Did you know... UTIs are the second most common type of infection in the body and more than half of all women experience at least one UTI during their lifetimes? Urinary tract infections are ten times more common among women than men.

Optimal Food/Nutrient Highlights

Cranberries, lingonberries, blueberries, horseradish, yogurt, kefir, cheese, vitamin C.

What Are Urinary Tract Infections?

Urinary tract infections can happen anywhere along the urinary tract. They occur when pathogenic bacteria adhere to the walls of the bladder, kidneys, ureters, or urethra and cause irritation. Most of the infections occur in the urethra and the bladder. Not everyone with a UTI has symptoms, but UTIs can become severe enough to warrant nearly 10 million doctor visits each year.

The most common symptoms include frequent urges to urinate with little urine expressed and a burning sensation in the bladder and/or urethra during urination. The urine may appear cloudy, milky, or reddish in color and may have an accompanying strong odor. Further progression of the infection to the kidneys can bring about a fever, feelings of nausea, and vomiting. Although most often an uncomfortable nuisance, left untreated, a UTI can lead to kidney infection and permanent damage.

A urine test that screens for bacteria and red blood cells is the most common way to test for a UTI.

What Causes UTIs?

Urinary tract infections are usually caused by the migration of *E. coli* bacteria, harmless (normally sterile) when they stay put in the colon, but troublesome when they cause contamination of the urinary system. Some people are more susceptible to getting UTIs than others. You could be at risk if you

Have an abnormality that obstructs the flow of urine such as a kidney stone or an enlarged prostate.

Have diabetes or immunosuppression.

Are sexually active, use a contraceptive method such as a diaphragm, or use spermicidal lubricants.

Have bowel incontinence.

Are immobile (for example, during recovery from a hip fracture).

Are in menopause.

Optimal Life Foods

Cranberries are one of the most researched foods for the treatment and prevention of UTIs. There are several studies that show that cranberries have antibacterial and antiadhesion properties (attributable to their proanthocyanidin and flavanol content). A review of ten studies that involved over 1,000 subjects demonstrated that cranberry juice may decrease symptomatic UTIs, especially in women with recurrent UTIs.

Special note: *People taking a blood-thinning medication such as Coumadin (warfarin) should avoid cranberry juice, as it may increase bleeding.*

Lingonberries. Trials have suggested cranberry and cranberry-lingonberry products to be beneficial in the prevention of UTIs.

Blueberries were shown in a study to have antiadhesive properties that may inhibit *E. coli* bacteria.

Horseradish. Several laboratory studies suggest that horseradish has antibiotic activity. One German study found that horseradish was as effective as standard antibiotic therapy.

Yogurt, kefir, and cheese. In a case-control study, women who ate yogurt and cheese or other fermented milk products more than three times a week were nearly 80 percent less likely to experience a urinary tract infection than women who ate them less than once a week.

Fluids. Despite the fact that science has yet to prove that drinking lots of fluids helps with UTIs, many health professionals recommend increased fluid intake. My own clinical experience has been that patients benefit from increased fluid intake.

Optimal Life Supplements

Vitamin C is a popular supplement for treating UTIs, as it is thought to acidify urine.

Uva ursi is an herb that has long been used as a folk remedy to treat UTIs. The active ingredients in the herb are ursolic acid and isoquercitrin, which inhibits bacterial growth and promotes urine flow.

Cranberry concentrate capsules. This is certainly an option for those who do not like the taste of cranberry juice or who like the convenience of taking a pill.

Caution! Calcium supplements. *Excess calcium in the urine may create an environment that makes it easier for bacteria to adhere to the walls of the urinary tract. However, in a case-control study, calcium from dairy products was not shown to increase UTI risk.*

Feeding the Fire!

Several foods are known to irritate the lining of the bladder or to contribute to the urge to urinate. If you are struggling with a UTI, consult with a registered dietitian about whether to avoid alcohol, spicy foods, coffee and other caffeinated beverages, acidy foods, citrus fruits and tomatoes, and chocolate.

UTI MENU PLAN

Day 1

Breakfast (375)
1 cup flaxseed cereal flakes (190)
1 cup skim milk (90)
½ cup cranberry juice (70)
1 teaspoon honey (25)
1 cup green tea

Lunch (530)
1 serving *Roasted Vegetable and Sweet Swiss Panini* (250)
(page 333)

1 serving *Zucchini-Cranberry Muffins* (190) (page 339)
1 cup skim milk (90)

Midday Snack (290)
1 serving *Chilean Fruit Guacamole* (100) (page 259)
12 fat-free corn chips (120)
½ cup cranberry juice (70)
1½ cups sparkling water with lime

Dinner (650)
4 ounces rotisserie chicken (220)
1 cup steamed Brussels sprouts (60)
1 serving *Polenta Pizza* (180) (page 329)
2 cups spinach salad with assorted veggies and citrus dressing
(120)
½ cup cranberry juice (70)
1 cup water

Evening Snack (234)
1 cup carrot sticks (50)
2 tablespoons hummus (54)
1 serving *Apple-Soy Chai Latte* (130) (page 254)

Day 2

Breakfast (420)
1 serving *Soufflé Omelet with Balsamic Strawberries* (160)
(page 345)
1 whole grain English muffin (100)
½ cup cranberry juice (70)
1 cup skim milk (90)

Lunch (590)

1 serving *Blackberry Smoothie* (320) (page 258)

1 serving *Mango-Tango Tilapia Salad* (270) (page 288)

Midday Snack (400)

1 serving *Rosemary Nuts* (290) (page 269)

4 ounces high-probiotic yogurt (110)

1 cup green tea

Dinner (674)

1 serving *Grilled Chicken Salad with Pomegranate Vinaigrette and Mango Gelée Garnish* (300) (page 324)

1 serving *Roasted Autumn Vegetables in Sherry Sauce* (114) (page 360)

1 whole grain roll (100)

½ cup cranberry juice (70)

1 cup skim milk (90)

Evening Snack (110)

1 serving *Beanie-Greenie Brownies* (110) (page 309)

1 cup decaffeinated green tea

Day 3

Breakfast (450)

1 serving *Georgia Pecan Muesli* (360) (page 344)

½ cup cranberry juice

1 cup skim milk (90)

Lunch (591)

1 serving *Raw Kale Salad with Lemon-Honey Vinaigrette* (260) (page 296)

1 serving *Chili-Honey Almond Chicken Kebabs* (261) (page 266)
½ cup cranberry juice (70)
1½ cups water with lemon

Midday Snack (230)
1 serving *Quick Pumpkin Smoothie* (230) (page 256)

Dinner (670)
1 serving *Mediterranean Grilled Mackerel or Bluefish*
(page 321) with 1 serving *Avocado Chimichurri* sauce
(page 300) (330)
1 serving *Watermelon and Feta Salad* (270) (page 294)
½ cup cranberry juice (70)
1½ cups water with lemon

Evening Snack (240)
1 serving *Spicy Biscotti* (130) (page 311)
4 ounces high-probiotic fruited yogurt (110)
1½ cups water with lemon

PART 6

A GOOD FOUNDATION

OSTEOPOROSIS AND OSTEOPENIA

Make No Bones About It

Did you know...*over 10 million Americans have osteoporosis and the costs associated with the disease are nearly $18 billion per year?*

Optimal Food/Nutrient Highlights

Yogurt, sardines, spinach, beans, mushrooms, fatty fish, onions, tea, soy, dried plums, vitamin B$_{12}$, calcium, vitamin D.

What Is Osteoporosis?

Osteoporosis (meaning "porous bones") is a disease in which bones lose density and become more fragile, increasing the risk of fracture. Rarely are there telltale signs of osteoporosis until painful fractures and breaks occur. The bones most vulnerable are the hip, spine, and wrist. Osteoporosis is also associated with higher mortality.

There are three general types of osteoporosis:

Type I (postmenopausal osteoporosis). This occurs in women over fifty, primarily due to a decrease in the hormones estrogen and androgen, which are responsible for maintaining bone density.

Type II (age-associated osteoporosis). Both women and men above sixty-five are at risk. Type II, more so than type I, is thought to be related to calcium and vitamin D deficiencies.

Idiopathic osteoporosis. Translated, it means no one has a clue why it happens. Adults and juveniles alike can be affected by this type. However, in juveniles' osteoporosis, it is most often reversible, as children continue to lay down bone well into their twenties. Like type I and type II, for adults, ideopathic osteoporosis cannot be reversed.

What Is Osteopenia?

Osteopenia describes bones that have lower mineral density than normal, but not nearly as severe as those with osteoporosis. Osteopenia most often leads to osteoporosis.

What Causes Osteoporosis and Osteopenia?

Type I Osteoporosis. Typically, women start off with less bone mass than men and tend to lose what they have more quickly due to the reduction in estrogen production as they age. So, between the ages of forty-five and fifty-five, when most women start menopause, estrogen production decreases, which causes calcium to leave the bones, making them more porous and brittle.

Type II Osteoporosis. Again, the bone density we retain when we get older depends on our peak bone mass in earlier years contrasted with the rate of loss. Factors that can influence the rate of loss are

- *Fractures that occur as an adult.*
- *Cigarette smoking.*
- *Low body weight or the opposite, obesity.*
- *Drug side effects.* Prednisone, heparin, and some antiseizure drugs can contribute to bone loss.
- *Medical challenges.* Gastric surgery, celiac disease, Crohn's disease, hyperparathyroidism, alcoholism, severe liver disease, and kidney failure affect calcium absorption.
- *Poor calcium and vitamin D intake.* As we age, the ability to synthesize vitamin D in the skin becomes lessened, and compounded with less sun exposure due to concerns of increased risk of skin cancer, adequate vitamin D intake becomes a challenge. Vitamin D helps calcium move into the bone, where it is needed.
- *Too little activity.* Not engaging in weight-bearing activities such as walking, running, dancing, and weight training.
- *Too much intense exercise,* such as marathon running, which can reduce estrogen levels.
- *Eating disorders or frequent dieting.* Both can reduce estrogen levels.

Optimal Life Foods

Calcium-rich foods. Considering that 98 percent of our calcium resides in the bones, it makes sense to include calcium food sources in our diets. Your best sources of calcium are listed below:

CALCIUM IN SELECTED FOODS

Yogurt, 1 cup: 415 mg

Sardines, in oil, drained, 3 ounces: 372 mg

Collard greens, cooked, 1 cup: 357 mg

Ricotta cheese, ⅓ cup: 337 mg

Nonfat milk, 1 cup: 302 mg

Pudding, vanilla, 1 cup: 298 mg

Whole milk, 1 cup: 291 mg

Custard, 1 cup: 297 mg.

Buttermilk, 1 cup: 286 mg

Ice milk, soft serve, 1 cup: 274 mg

Swiss cheese, 1 ounce: 272 mg

Turnip greens, cooked, 1 cup: 249 mg

Rhubarb, cooked, 1 cup: 212 mg

Spinach, cooked, 1 cup: 200 mg

Refried beans, canned, 1 cup: 141 mg

Vitamin D–rich foods enhance the absorption of calcium into the bones. Food sources include mushrooms, egg yolks, and fatty fish.

DASH (dietary approaches to stopping hypertension) diet. DASH is probably one of my favorite dietary programs. It is a standout for osteoporosis—a calcium-rich diet that emphasizes fruits, vegetables, and low-fat dairy products. Besides being great for controlling blood pressure, this diet pulls together a variety of bone-promoting foods from lean meats to whole grains, low-fat dairy products, fruits, and vegetables. An intervention study that included a variety of different-aged men and women showed that a diet like the DASH diet, which is high in fruits and vegetables and low-fat dairy products, had a profound effect on reducing bone turnover. Carotenes are found extensively in fruits and vegetables, and these nutrients have been shown to be important to the skeleton. Several population-based studies published between 2001 and 2006 demonstrated the beneficial effects on bone parameters from consuming fruits and vegetables for men and women of all ages. The nutrients found in abundance in fruits and vegetables were shown to improve bone mass and markers of bone resorption. Specifically, those women who had the lowest intake of potassium, magnesium, fiber, vitamin C, and beta-carotene had significantly lower spine and neck bone mineral density (BMD).

Onions. Scientists at the University of Bern found a peptide compound in onions called GPCS that slowed down bone loss in an animal study.

Tea. One would think that tea, with its caffeine and oxalates, would not be a good idea to consume if you wanted to preserve bone mass. Wrong! A study in 2007 found that elderly women who drank tea had better hip preservation than non–tea drinkers.

Soy. The research available on the effects of soy alone on bone health is mixed. Much of it looks at isolating estrogen-like compounds and evaluating their effects on bone. But interestingly, there are studies that show when soy protein and omega-3 fats are combined in the diet, they exert an anti-inflammatory effect that slows down osteoclastic (bone breakdown) activity. Eating whole soy foods provides both the protein and omega-3 fats.

Dried plums. Insulin-like growth factor 1 (IGF-1) has a powerful effect on increasing bone mineral density. Consuming dried plums was found to increase the level of IGF-1 in postmenopausal women. An animal study looked at the effect of combining soy protein, dried plums, and fructooligosaccharides (FOS) on lumbar bone mineral density and found it to be the more pronounced effect compared with a soy protein or casein diet alone in increasing lumbar BMD.

Optimal Life Supplements

Vitamin B_{12}. In the first large-scale study, involving more than 2,500 men and women, researchers from Tufts University found that those who had low levels of B_{12} also had lower-than-average bone density. Vitamin B_{12} mainly comes from animal proteins and fortified foods in the diet.

Calcium and vitamin D. For most adults challenged with osteoporosis or osteopenia, a daily intake of between 1,200 and 1,500 mg of calcium and at least 1,000 IU of vitamin D is both safe and effective. Calcium supplements appear to be most effective in reducing bone loss in women who are at least five years postmenopause, especially those who have also had poor calcium intake. In women who are less than five years postmenopausal and are not vitamin D deficient, calcium supplementation has shown little effect on bone mineral density. Results of randomized, controlled trials are mixed, and the effects of vitamin D supplementation on calcium absorption in children has not been studied.

Feeding the Fire!

A diet that is lacking in calcium, potassium, and vitamin D and is too rich in protein, sodium, and caffeine may have negative effects on bone health. With this in mind, you may consider limiting the following:

Cola beverages. It used to be the assumption that high carbonated beverage consumption increased urinary calcium excretion, but that is debatable according to the scientific literature. However, in the Framingham Osteoporosis Study (a food-questionnaire study), there was a correlation between drinking cola and lower bone-mineral density. Bottom line: If you like cola beverages, proceed with caution (for now).

Excess fiber. Excessive fiber intake has been shown to interfere with calcium absorption. Of course, the likelihood of that happening for the average American is pretty slim given that our average fiber intake is pretty abysmal. As long as you are not exceeding the recommended levels of twenty-five to thirty-five grams, you should be in good shape.

Excess protein. High-protein diets have demonstrated increased urinary calcium losses—one of the reasons I'm not a big fan of them. Animal protein consumed in large quantities increases urinary losses of calcium compared with plant sources of protein like soy.

Excess salt. High sodium intake increases urinary calcium excretion. And a high-sodium diet is often a double whammy because it is almost always accompanied by low potassium intake.

Chocolate. Although chocolate is rich in the types of flavonoids that may help with bone health, there is some research that has shown that older women who consume chocolate daily have lower bone density and strength. Chocolate contains oxalates, which can impact calcium absorption. Bottom line: Enjoy in moderation.

BONE-BUILDING MENU PLAN

Day 1

Breakfast (360)
1 serving *Creamy Cherry Oatmeal* (210) (page 350)
1 cup skim milk (90)
½ cup orange juice (calcium and vitamin D fortified) (60)

Lunch (530)
1 serving *Roasted Vegetable and Sweet Swiss Panini* (250) (page 333)
1 ounce whole grain pretzels (110)
½ cup pomegranate juice (80)
1 cup skim milk (90)

Midday Snack (250)
2 servings *Royal Blue Cheese–Stuffed Mushrooms* (120) (page 260)
1 serving *Apple-Soy Chai Latte* (130) (page 254)

Dinner (730)
4 ounces rotisserie chicken (220)
1 serving *Curried Chickpeas and Kale* (150) (page 370)
1 serving *Grilled Vidalia Onion and Peach Salad* (270) (page 292)
1 cup skim milk (90)

Evening Snack (140)
1 serving *Christine's Baked Custard* (140) (page 308)
1 cup decaffeinated green tea

Day 2

Breakfast (360)
1 serving *Creamy Cherry Oatmeal* (210) (page 350)
½ cup orange juice (calcium and vitamin D fortified) (60)
1 cup skim milk (90)

Lunch (480)
1 serving *Christine's Yummy Bean and Cheese Tostada* (260)
(page 319)
1 serving *Avocado-Fennel Citrus Salad* (120) (page 285)
4 to 5 dried plums (100)
1 cup green tea

Midday Snack (370)
1 serving *Sardine Salad / Dip* (320) (page 265)
1 cup carrot and celery sticks (50)
1 cup green tea

Dinner (694)
2 servings *Kale Balls* (80) (page 262)
1 serving *Chicken Thighs with Red Wine, Dried Plums, and
Garlic* (310) (page 323)
1 serving *Roasted Autumn Vegetables in Sherry Sauce* (114)
(page 360)
1 whole grain roll (100)
1 cup skim milk (90)

Evening Snack (110)
1 serving *Beanie-Greenie Brownies* (110) (page 309)
1 cup decaffeinated green tea

Day 3

Breakfast (325)
1 serving *Raspberry-Yogurt Muffins* (160) (page 338)
1 cup fruited yogurt (110)
½ cup diced mango (55)
1 cup green tea

Lunch (443)
1 serving *Healthy Turkey Salad Pocket* (233) (page 335)
1 serving *Sharon's Moroccan Couscous* (210) (page 359)
1½ cups water with lemon

Midday Snack (196)
1 serving *Asian Satay Skewers with Black Bean Sauce* (196)
(page 263)
1½ cups water with lemon

Dinner (700)
1 serving *Garlic Pipérade Soup* (150) (page 274)
1 serving *Irish Poached Salmon* (350) (page 320)
1 serving *Sicilian Broccoli Salad* (200) (page 291)
1 cup decaffeinated green tea

Evening snack (290)
1 serving *Powerhouse Dried Plum Bars* (200) (page 343)
1 cup skim milk (90)

Dr. Christine Gerbstadt's Top Ten Tips for Fighting Osteoporosis

Christine Gerbstadt, MD, RD, is a national spokesperson for the American Dietetic Association and founder of the Nutronics Health program (www.NutronicsHealth.com).

1. *Eat a calcium- and vitamin-rich diet.* Include at least three servings per day of calcium-rich and vitamin D–fortified dairy such as nonfat milk and yogurt, or calcium- and vitamin D–fortified orange juice, and whole grain cereals. Food sources of vitamin D include vitamin D–fortified milk and soy milk (400 IU per quart), fortified cereals (40–50 IU per serving), egg yolks, saltwater fish, and liver.
2. *Limit total caffeine* to no more than two cups of coffee or equivalent caffeine per day.
3. *Reduce alcohol intake* to no more than three drinks per day or twenty-one per week.
4. *Take calcium and vitamin D supplements.* Aim for 1,200 mg of calcium and 800–1,000 IU of vitamin D per day for adults aged fifty and older. Low calcium intake and vitamin D insufficiency increase a person's risk for osteoporosis.
5. *Consult with your doctor if you are on the following substances,* which can worsen osteoporosis or increase your risk:

   - Oral glucocorticoids such as prednisone. Five milligrams or more per day taken for three months at any point in time will increase a person's risk for osteoporosis.
   - Vitamin A supplements (nonfood sources).
   - Aluminum salts found in antacids.

6. *Consider medication.* Postmenopausal women should discuss the current FDA-approved pharmacologic options for osteoporosis management with their doctor.

- *Bisphosphonates (alendronate, ibandronate, risedronate, and zoledronic acid)* may cause stomach upset and inflammation and erosions of the esophagus, which can be reduced by remaining seated upright for thirty to sixty minutes after taking the medication.
- *Calcitonin* may be associated with nausea and vomiting.
- *Estrogens* and/or hormone therapy.
- *Parathyroid hormone (teriparatide).*
- *Estrogen agonist/antagonist (raloxifene).*

There are no specific food or supplement interactions for the above drugs.

7. *Enjoy adequate weight-bearing exercise,* where bones and muscles work against gravity as the lower extremities bear the body's weight, such as walking, jogging, tai chi, stair climbing, dancing, and tennis, and adequate muscle-strengthening exercise such as weight training and other resistive exercises at least three times a week.
8. *Stop smoking* and do not be around secondhand smoke.
9. *Reduce fall risk* with environmental modifications such as removing loose area rugs, and with gait and balance training. Get a dual-energy X-ray absorptiometry (DXA) measurement by age sixty-five for women and seventy for men, and evaluate U.S. fracture risk algorithm (FRAX) risk.
10. *Consider gaining weight* if your body mass index is below 19. Get treatment if you have an eating disorder.

ARTHRITIS

A Royal Pain

Did you know . . . *a type of arthritis called gout was at one time in history considered socially desirable because of its prevalence among the elite? Although quite painful, because of gout's association with a more affluent lifestyle, it has often been referred to as the disease of kings.*

Optimal Food/Nutrient Highlights

Avocados, soy, omega-3s, antioxidants, olive oil, cooked vegetables, ginger, Mediterranean diet, vitamin C, vitamin D, low-fat dairy products, coffee, wine, tart cherries, garlic, fiber, folate.

What Is Arthritis?

According to the Centers for Disease Control and Prevention, approximately one-quarter of American adults have been diagnosed with arthritis. The term *arthritis* refers to more than 100 different diseases that, according to the Arthritis Foundation, cause "pain, stiffness, and sometimes swelling in or around joints."

Osteoarthritis (OA) is the most common form of arthritis and is a degenerative joint disease in which the cartilage in the joint deteriorates, causing pain and loss of movement.

Rheumatoid arthritis (RA) is less common than OA and involves autoimmune and inflammatory processes at the joints, causing swelling and progressive joint damage. Osteoarthritis occurs mostly in the elderly; however, RA onset is most common in middle age and even in young adults.

Gout is one of the oldest known and most common forms of arthritis, dating back to the Egyptians in 2640 BC. It is the most common inflammatory arthritis in adult men in Western countries but is rapidly becoming more evident among older women. The occurrence of gout in the United States has approximately doubled over the past two decades.

What Causes Arthritis?

Osteoarthritis. Although the cause is not known, it may be a combination of factors such as heredity, prior injury to the joint, obesity, and the natural aging process.

Rheumatoid arthritis is an autoimmune disorder and the cause is unknown.

Gout has been associated throughout history with rich foods and excessive alcohol consumption. It is attributed to the accumulation of monosodium urate crystals in the joint, which causes pain. High serum uric acid levels, also known as hyperuricemia, are thought to be the result of a combination of factors such as a high-purine diet, alcohol use, diuretic therapy, and poor kidney function. What differentiates gout from other forms of arthritis is the detection of monosodium urate crystals in the synovial fluid of the joint upon diagnosis.

Optimal Life Foods

Osteoarthritis

Cherries. In a study reported in *The Journal of Nutrition,* supplementing the diets of healthy men and women with cherries reduced markers of inflammation.

Avocados and soy. Two studies of avocados and soybeans showed beneficial effects on pain in osteoarthritis patients.

Vitamin D. Higher blood levels of vitamin D have been associated with improved muscle strength and physical function and less pain in subjects with osteoarthritis of the knee. Besides sunlight, dietary sources of vitamin D include fortified margarine, oily fish, liver, fortified breakfast cereals, mushrooms, and dairy products.

Rheumatoid Arthritis

Omega-3s and antioxidants. Rheumatoid arthritis patients should consume a balanced diet rich in long-chain n-3 polyunsaturated fatty acids (PUFAs) and antioxidants for best control of pain and inflammation.

Olive oil and cooked vegetables. Consumption of both vegetables and olive oil was associated with a lower risk of RA in a large study.

Ginger. Research involving persons with OA and RA has provided limited evidence that ginger may reduce arthritic pain, but a recent animal study showed significant reduction in joint swelling using a crude extract of ginger versus a standardized extract. This suggests that ginger has benefits beyond its known gingerol components.

A *Mediterranean diet,* characterized by a high consumption of fruits, vegetables, whole grains, and legumes, a reduced intake of meat, and more intake of fish, has been reported to decrease inflammation of arthritis.

Vitamin C–rich foods. In a study featured in the *Annals of the Rheumatic Diseases,* people who ate the least amount of vitamin C–rich fruits and vegetables were twice as likely to develop inflammation in the joints compared with those who ate the most. Vitamin C–rich foods include citrus fruits, strawberries, and red bell peppers.

Gout

Weight management. There is growing evidence that a calorie-restricted and lower-refined-carbohydrate diet is more effective in treating gout than the conventional low-purine diet. Insulin resistance seems to be more of an issue than thought previously, so targeting fat around the gut would be of benefit.

Low-fat dairy products were shown to help control uric acid effects.

Coffee (but not tea) intake was associated with lower levels of uric acid (a common aggravator of gout) in the blood.

Wine. Although certain alcoholic beverages seem to aggravate gout, wine does not appear to be one of them. Wine drinkers tend to have lower uric acid levels, which is thought to be due to the protective effect of antioxidants in wine, or possibly better diet and lifestyle choices in general of wine drinkers, or both.

Tart cherries were shown to lower urate in the blood in one small study.

Vegetable protein from wheat gluten was found helpful in lowering urate levels in a study conducted by David Jenkins, MD, PhD, DSc.

Dietary fiber, folate, and vitamin C, as found in a variety of fruits and vegetables, help protect against hyperuricemia and gout.

GLA and omega-3 fats. Animal research suggests that diets featuring gamma-linolenic acid (GLA) and omega-3 fats, especially eicosapentaenoic acid (EPA), can decrease inflammation associated with gout. Their effect on humans is still under study.

Garlic has been used widely for controlling gout.

Soy. Although tofu and other soy products are considered high-purine foods, most of the purines are lost during the processing of soybean products, and soy has been found to have only marginal negative effects, if any, in gout sufferers.

Optimal Life Supplements

Osteoarthritis

Ginger. Besides the root form used in cooking, ginger also comes in capsule form and is an effective anti-inflammatory.

Curcumin is an active component of turmeric and has wonderful anti-inflammatory properties.

Vitamin D. Low intake and low serum levels of vitamin D each appear to be associated with an increased risk for progression of osteoarthritis of the knee.

Glucosamine and chondroitin appear to be well tolerated and seem to provide modest benefits for persons with OA. Because persons with RA have some symptoms of OA, these supplements may be beneficial for RA as well.

Methylsulfonylmethane (MSM) has been shown to decrease pain in individuals with osteoarthritis.

Devil's claw. Studies of persons with OA of the knee have provided limited but promising evidence that devil's claw (Harpagophytum extract) reduces musculoskeletal pain.

Rheumatoid Arthritis

Vitamin D_3. Plasma levels of vitamin D_3 have been found to be inversely correlated with RA.

Gamma-linolenic acid (GLA) (evening primrose oil and borage oil). Several studies have found improvement in relief of pain, morning stiffness, and joint tenderness when RA subjects supplemented with GLA. This herbal intervention may provide supplementary or alternative treatment to NSAIDs for some patients.

Fish oil and olive oil. Forty-three patients with RA showed greater improvement in their symptoms when fish oil supplements were used in combination with olive oil.

Conjugated linoleic acid has been shown to exhibit anti-inflammatory activity.

Vitamin E has been found effective in reducing pain in subjects who have RA.

Selenium. In a double-blind, randomized-control trial, subjects who took selenium supplements reported a significant decrease in RA symptoms, reduced reliance on medication for managing symptoms, and a significant decrease in markers of inflammation. However, both the supplementation group and the placebo group received fish oil, so it is difficult to tell if the positive effect is attributable to selenium alone.

Gout

Garlic.

Folic acid. Some research has shown a beneficial effect of high-dose supplementation on serum urate levels, while another study showed no effect on reducing urate levels.

Caution! *Many doctors suggest taking vitamin C as a way to reduce uric acid, which might benefit gout. However, taking large amounts of vitamin C could also abruptly change urate levels in the* *blood, triggering a gout attack. One study showed that long-term use of vitamin C supplements might aggravate osteoarthritis.*

Feeding the Fire!

Osteoarthritis

A few years ago, my father called me in the middle of the night complaining of excruciating back pain. I immediately took him to the emergency room, where it was discovered that he had profuse osteoarthritis of the spine. His doctors offered him painkillers and suggested that surgery might be in his future. He asked me if I knew of any dietary intervention or supplements that might work. I had a smattering of experience with a nightshade-free diet with a few of my arthritis patients and thought I would propose it to him. "What? Have you forgotten that we are Italian?" pointed out my dad. Apparently, I had cut him to the quick with that advice; nonetheless, he was willing to try it. Within a matter of days of giving up tomatoes, potatoes, eggplant, and peppers, my father was pain-free—not a reduction in pain, mind you, but a complete elimination of pain! He was obviously a "positive responder" to the nightshade-free diet. A few short weeks later, I found my dad complaining once again about his arthritis pain—not as badly as the time we took the trip to the hospital, though. He relayed to me that in fact, he had added many of the foods back into his diet that I had asked him to avoid. Complete avoidance of his favorite foods was not going to happen anymore and it was worth a little pain and suffering to once again be able to enjoy them. For my dad, the "cure" was worse than the condition!

Nightshades. In a few studies, plants in the nightshade family, Solanaceae, have been found to cause pain and swelling in a small population of subjects with degenerative arthritis. Unfortunately, there isn't a way to test for nightshade sensitivity. The only way to know is to totally eliminate members of the nightshade family, which include potatoes (not sweet potatoes), tomatoes, eggplant, peppers (all varieties except black), and tobacco.

Rheumatoid Arthritis

Red meat. A trial of 25,000 men and women found that those who had the highest level of red meat consumption had a twofold risk of rheumatoid arthritis. Small studies have found a positive response to following a gluten-free vegan diet (no animal products) in RA patients.

The exclusion of foods such as citrus, chocolate, alcohol, and spices has led to inconsistent results, but might be worth a try.

Gout

Purines and animal proteins. Though a low-purine diet has been the standard of care for years, research to date has been unable to support total protein intake or consumption of purine-rich foods in association with increased risk of gout. However, high red meat intake has been associated with gout flare-ups.

Seafood.

Alcohol (especially beer and spirits). Wine does not have the same effect.

Sugar-sweetened soft drinks.

High-fructose fruits such as apples and oranges.

Diuretic foods. These include caffeine (over three cups of coffee a day, tea [especially green tea], colas), cranberry juice, asparagus, celery, eggplant, lemons, garlic, cucumbers, and licorice.

ANTI-ARTHRITIS MENU PLAN

Day 1

Breakfast (325)
1 cup flaxseed cereal flakes (190)
1 cup skim milk (90)
½ cup tart cherries (45)
1 cup coffee

Lunch (659)
1 serving *Asian Satay Skewers with Black Bean Sauce* (196) (page 263)
1 serving *Tropical Fruit and Shrimp Gazpacho* (80) (page 279)
1 serving *Cherry Zinger Smoothie* (383) (page 256)

Midday Snack (240)
1 serving *Beanie-Greenie Brownies* (110) (page 309)
1 serving *Apple-Soy Chai Latte* (130) (page 254)

Dinner (640)
4 ounces grilled chicken (220)
1 serving *Polenta Pizza* (180) (page 329)
2 cups spinach salad with olive oil and balsamic vinegar (120)
1 cup coffee
5 ounces red wine (optional) (120)

Evening Snack (180)
1 serving *Cheese-and-Fruit Kebabs* (70) (page 272)
1 serving *Super Fruit Relish* (110) (page 304)
1 cup herbal tea

Day 2

Breakfast (350)
1 serving *Soufflé Omelet with Balsamic Strawberries* (160)
(page 345)
1 whole grain English muffin (100)
1 cup skim milk (90)
1 cup coffee

Lunch (458)
1 cup pasta with 2 tablespoons pesto sauce (288)
1 serving *Avocado-Fennel Citrus Salad* (120) (page 285)
1 cup strawberries (50)
1 cup coffee

Midday Snack (310)
1 serving *"Devils on Horseback"* (180) (page 270)
1 serving *Apple-Soy Chai Latte* (130) (page 254)

Dinner (590)
1 serving *Winter Squash Soup with Roasted Seeds* (70)
(page 277)
1 serving *Irish Poached Salmon* (350) (page 320)
1 serving *Asparagus-Sesame Stir-Fry* (100) (page 362)
½ cup cherry juice (70)
1 cup herbal tea

Evening Snack (210)
1 serving *Asparagus-Carrot Rolls* (210) (page 361)
1½ cups water

Day 3

Breakfast (573)
1 serving *Triple-Grain Georgia Pecan Pancakes* (188)
(page 346)
2 scrambled omega-3 eggs with 1 slice cheese (250)
½ cup tart cherries (45)
1 cup skim milk (90)
1 cup coffee

Lunch (500)
1 serving *Mango-Tango Tilapia Salad* (270) (page 288)
1 whole grain roll (100)
1 serving *Strawberry-Papaya Smoothie* (130) (page 255)
1 cup coffee

Midday Snack (220/240)
1 serving *Spicy Biscotti* (130) (page 311)
1 cup skim or light soy milk (90/110)

Dinner (690)
1 serving *Mediterranean Grilled Mackerel or Bluefish* (250)
(page 321)
1 serving *Bean-Corn Salad* (120) (page 290)
1 serving *Quinoa Pilaf with Currants and Turmeric* (320)
(page 369)
1 cup herbal tea

Evening Snack (140)
1 serving *Cheese-and-Fruit Kebabs* (70) (page 272)
½ cup cherry juice (70)

Dave's Tips

1. Tai chi improves range of motion of the ankle, hip, and knee in people with rheumatoid arthritis.
2. Get movin'! Both high-intensity and low-intensity aerobic exercise reduces pain and improves functional status, gait, and aerobic capacity for people with OA of the knee.
3. Achieve a healthy weight. According to the Centers for Disease Control and Prevention, the prevalence of arthritis increases as weight does. Maintaining a healthy weight can help prevent arthritis and slow the progression of the disease.
4. Stay hydrated. Dehydration can cause elevated uric acid. Hydration is recommended as part of a treatment program for gout.
5. Eat regularly. Don't skip meals! Fasting is also associated with elevated uric acid in gout. Also, don't drink on an empty stomach—the combination of fasting and alcohol has a devastating effect on uric acid metabolism.
6. Take a chronic pain class. The Arthritis Foundation and some medical centers have classes for people with osteoarthritis or chronic pain. Ask your doctor about classes in your area or check with the Arthritis Foundation (www.arthritis.org). These classes teach skills that help you manage your osteoarthritis pain. And you'll meet other people with osteoarthritis and learn their tips for reducing joint pain or coping with your type of pain.
7. Focus on fiber! Fruits, vegetables, and whole grains have protective effects against hyperuricemia and gout.

DEGENERATIVE DISC DISEASE (DDD)

Give It the Slip

Did you know...*more than 65 million Americans experience back pain each year and more than 85 percent of the population will have degenerative disc disease (DDD) by the age of fifty? Most who have the condition don't even know they have it, but for those who do know, it can be quite painful.*

Optimal Food/Nutrient Highlights

Fluids, fatty fish, walnuts, hemp, flaxseed, soy, canola oil, mushrooms, cherries, avocados, soy, curcumin, vitamin D, calcium.

What Is Degenerative Disc Disease?

This health challenge is near and dear to my heart...or should I say neck? I was diagnosed with this condition a few years ago and found it to be quite painful (my discs were herniated, to boot). Degenerative disc disease is not really a "disease," but rather is a general term to describe deterioration of what are called intervertebral discs that run throughout the spine. The intervertebral discs are fibrous and jellylike and separate the vertebrae. They act as "shock absorbers" and enable the spine to flex. As you age, the discs begin to dehydrate, causing them to shrink and stiffen. The end result is the loss of flexibility and narrowing of the space that separates the vertebrae. This combination can often result in back pain.

Though my DDD occurred in my neck, it often presents in the

lower-back area known as the lumbar region. Besides pain and limitation of movement, degenerative disc disease can also result in

Bone spurs (osteophytes). Protruding abnormal bone growth between the joints that can cause pain.

A herniated disc. Rupturing of a disc, placing increased pressure on nerves that run down the spinal cord.

Osteoarthritis. The deterioration of cartilage between the joints.

Spinal stenosis. A narrowing of the opening that the spinal cord runs through.

What Causes Degenerative Disc Disease?

Live long enough, and odds are you will develop DDD. The majority of cases are simply attributed to the wear and tear of daily living and considered a natural part of aging. However, more and more people in their earlier years, even in their twenties, are developing DDD, suggesting that there may be other factors at play.

Obesity. Rising rates of obesity have been attributed to additional stress and strain on the infrastructure of the body.

Injury. Degenerative disc disease can occur after a traumatic injury to the spine.

Occupation. Heavy lifting, especially when stomach muscles are weak, can contribute to lumbar DDD. More cervical cases of DDD have been associated with continued neck strain during an activity such as working on the computer for hours on end.

Heredity.

Cigarette smoking increases spinal disc degeneration by 20 percent, according to research. Blood vessels that feed the discs constrict from smoking.

Osteoporosis.

Arthritis.

Low vitamin D and/or calcium levels. Low levels may lead to osteoarthritis and subject the spine and discs to disease progression.

Optimal Life Foods

Drink plenty of fluids. Joints need fluid, too!

Fatty fish. Consume two 3-ounce servings of fish rich in the omega-3 fatty acids per week to help decrease inflammation. Salmon, mackerel, sardines, and albacore tuna are all good sources.

Walnuts, hemp, flaxseed, soy (and their oils), and canola oil. These foods are rich in the omega-3 fatty acid alpha-linolenic acid, which is important in helping to decrease inflammation, and are good vegetarian choices.

Vitamin D and calcium. Vitamin D–fortified milk or soy milk, fortified orange juice, and yogurt may increase bone density. (In a study conducted by T. E. McAlindon and colleagues, a threefold increase in the risk of osteoarthritis progression was found for patients with the middle and lowest levels of serum 25–hydroxy vitamin D.)

Mushrooms contain about 16 IU of vitamin D in a standard serving of four or five mushrooms. But Penn State researchers discovered that when mushrooms were exposed to ultraviolet light one hour before harvesting, the vitamin D content of the mushrooms got kicked up to twice the FDA daily value—800 IU! And when the mushrooms were exposed to ultraviolet rays after harvesting, the vitamin D quadrupled in daily value! Vitamin D purists always recommend animal-source vitamin D_3, but research suggests the vitamin D_2 found in mushrooms is absorbed very well and can help retain calcium in the spine.

Optimal Life Supplements

A multivitamin with antioxidants. Treatment with antioxidants in the initial stages of DDD may be useful as secondary therapy to prevent the oxidative damage to and deterioration of the musculoskeletal tissues in osteoarthritis.

Glucosamine and chondroitin in some studies were found to be a safe alternative to NSAIDs.

Avocado/soybean unsaponifiables may help reduce the need for NSAIDs, as they appear to help decrease inflammation and stimulate cartilage repair. In France, avocado/soybean unsaponifiables have been approved as a prescription drug.

The proteolytic enzyme bromelain, the protein-digestive enzyme found in pineapple, reduces inflammation.

Cherry extract is probably the number one supplement I depended on to help control pain when my DDD flared up!

Fish oil helps reduce inflammatory prostaglandins.

Curcumin is the naturally occurring plant chemical found in the Indian spice turmeric. Studies have found that taking curcumin along with NSAIDs increases their effectiveness up to tenfold! Like unsaponifiables, curcumin may decrease the need for NSAIDs.

Caution! *Patients on blood thinners should be careful taking chondroitin, as it can increase the blood thinning and cause excessive bleeding.*

Feeding the Fire!

Research has shown that raising the intake of omega-3 fats aids the body in producing helpful anti-inflammatory prostaglandins that may benefit DDD. However, Americans consume substantially more omega-6-variety than omega-3 fats, and some have theorized that this skewed balance may result in an overproduction of in-flammatory prostaglandins. You should consider limiting—not necessarily eliminating—safflower oil (high-oleic versions are bet-ter to use), corn oil, sunflower oil, and animal fat.

DDD MENU PLAN

Day 1

Breakfast (380)
1 cup flaxseed cereal flakes (190)
1 cup skim milk (90)
4 to 5 dried plums (100)
1 cup green tea

Lunch (570)
1 serving *Roasted Vegetable and Sweet Swiss Panini* (250) (page 333)
1 serving *Blackberry Smoothie* (320) (page 258)

Midday Snack (290)
1 serving *Rosemary Nuts* (290) (page 269)
1 cup green tea

Dinner (660)
4 ounces rotisserie chicken (220)
1 serving *Nuts and Berry Fruit Salad* (350) (page 286)
1 cup skim milk (90)

Evening Snack (200)
1 serving *Powerhouse Dried Plum Bars* (200) (page 343)
1 cup decaffeinated green tea

Day 2

Breakfast (480)
1 serving *Soufflé Omelet with Balsamic Strawberries* (160)
(page 345)
1 serving *Spicy Biscotti* (130) (page 311)
1 whole grain English muffin (100)
1 cup skim milk (90)
1 cup green tea

Lunch (440)
1 serving *Blackberry Smoothie* (320) (page 258)
1 serving *Avocado-Fennel Citrus Salad* (120) (page 285)

Midday Snack (290)
1 serving *Rosemary Nuts* (290) (page 269)
1 cup green tea

Dinner (694)
1 serving *Cocoa-Encrusted Salmon with Blueberries* (270)
(page 330)
1 serving *Roasted Autumn Vegetables in Sherry Sauce* (114)
(page 360)

2 servings *Royal Blue Cheese–Stuffed Mushrooms* (120) (page 260)
1 whole grain roll (100)
1 cup skim milk (90)

Evening Snack (110)
1 serving *Beanie-Greenie Brownies* (110) (page 309)
1 cup decaffeinated green tea

Day 3

Breakfast (463)
1 serving *Triple-Grain Georgia Pecan Pancakes* (188) (page 346)
1 turkey sausage link (140)
½ cup tart cherries (45)
1 cup skim milk (90)

Lunch (440)
1 serving *Tropical Fruit and Shrimp Gazpacho* (80) (page 279)
1 serving *Raw Kale Salad with Lemon-Honey Vinaigrette* (260) (page 296)
1 whole grain roll (100)
1½ cups water with lemon

Midday Snack (130)
1 serving *Strawberry-Papaya Smoothie* (130) (page 255)

Dinner (646)
1 serving *Chicken Thighs with Red Wine, Dried Plums, and Garlic* (310) (page 323)
1 serving *Sicilian Broccoli Salad* (200) (page 291)

½ cup brown rice (100)

1 serving *Watermelon Soda* (36) (page 253)

Evening Snack (390)

1 serving *Summer Fruits Pie* (390) (page 315)

1 cup decaffeinated green tea

Dave's Tips

1. Take a break from the computer. Bending over for extended periods of time is hard on the back!
2. Yoga and Pilates may benefit you, but seek the guidance of a health professional.

PART 7

EYES ON THE FUTURE

AGE-RELATED MACULAR DEGENERATION (AMD) AND CATARACTS

Look Out!

Did you know . . . *macular degeneration is the leading cause of irreversible blindness in persons over sixty-five in the United States? Over 3.5 million Americans over the age of forty are blind or have low vision, with this number projected to rise to 5.5 million by 2020. According to AMD Alliance International, age-related macular degeneration (AMD) affects more than 30 million people worldwide aged fifty or over.*

Optimal Food/Nutrient Highlights

Corn, egg yolks, spinach, pistachios, avocados, goji berries, lutein, zeaxanthin, vitamin A/beta-carotene, vitamin E, omega-3 fats.

I have grouped macular degeneration and cataracts together because their dietary interventions for prevention and treatment are virtually identical. The emphasis here is really on prevention. If you have the beginning stages of either macular degeneration or cataracts, following the diet and lifestyle recommendations contained here alone may be quite helpful in slowing down the process.

What Is Age-Related Macular Degeneration?

Age-related macular degeneration is a progressive disease process that causes damage to the macula—part of the retina portion of the eye—which is responsible for acute vision. The end result is gradual erosion of the central vision of the eye. Age-related macular degeneration can occur in one or both of the eyes.

Types of AMD

Dry AMD
This variety is more common, accounting for 85 to 90 percent of all cases of AMD. In dry AMD, there is an accumulation of a substance called drusen, which are tiny white to yellowish spots caused by the accumulation of debris from the deteriorating retina. The accumulation of drusen alone does not usually cause vision loss.

The Three Stages of Dry AMD
Early: The appearance of several small- to medium-sized drusen. Generally there are no symptoms.

Intermediate: The appearance of several medium- or one or more large-sized drusen. A "blurred" spot in the center of vision may appear.

Advanced: Several drusen appear plus breakdown of cells in the macula region. The "blurred" spot appears bigger and darker.

Wet AMD

Wet AMD develops from the dry form of AMD. The wet form is referred to as neovascular, because there is growth of new blood vessels in the area of the macula. It is the more serious form of the two because the blood vessels that grow beneath the retina eventually cause hemorrhaging, swelling, and the formation of scar tissue. The end result is permanent damage that creates blind spots in the central vision.

What Causes Age-Related Macular Degeneration?

There are many risk factors for AMD. The first four listed below contribute to oxidative stress on the macula and may be considered "modifiable" risk factors. Although nothing can be done about chronological aging, your lifestyle choices most certainly can slow down biological aging!

Aging.

Diabetes.

Smoking.

Obesity.

Cardiovascular risk factors, including controlled and uncontrolled hypertension and elevated inflammatory markers such as C-reactive protein (CRP) and interleukin-6 (IL-6).

Race (Caucasians).

Family history (genetics).

Gender (women).

What Are Cataracts?

Cataracts are abnormally clumped proteins that occur in the lens portion of the eye and cause "clouded" vision. The majority of cataracts are associated with the aging process and can occur in one or both eyes. The clumped proteins give a yellowish to brownish cast to the lens.

What Causes Cataracts?

Most cataracts are due to the aging process, but they can also be brought about by smoking, alcohol abuse, diseases such as diabetes and glaucoma, prolonged exposure to the sun, congenital defects, and exposure to certain types of radiation.

Optimal Life Foods

Observational studies indicate that diets that are rich in fruits and vegetables (especially the yellow and leafy green varieties) help decrease the risk of AMD and cataracts.

Lutein and zeaxanthin. These plant chemicals are highly concentrated in the macula and work as potent antioxidants that protect eyes from free radical damage. Eating foods that are high in lutein and zeaxanthin, such as dark green leafy vegetables, yellow fruits and yellow vegetables such as corn, and egg yolks has been found to reduce the risk of cataracts by up to 20 percent and AMD risk by up to 40 percent. Other optimal life food sources include avocados, pistachios, goji berries, orange bell peppers, kiwis, grapes, spinach, orange juice, squash (zucchini), kale, collard greens, Brussels sprouts, and green beans.

Vitamin A/beta-carotene, in foods such as carrots, apricots, romaine lettuce, and broccoli.

Vitamin E–rich foods such as almonds and whole grains.

Omega-3 fats. A study in *The American Journal of Clinical Nutrition* found that eating fatty fish like salmon, mackerel, and tuna— just once a week—may reduce the risk of AMD by as much as 50 percent. And if fatty fish is consumed more than once a week, the risk of wet AMD may be reduced by as much as 70 percent! Other omega-3 sources include eggs that are omega-3 enriched, walnuts, canola oil, and flaxseed.

Optimal Life Supplements

A multivitamin. Look for a formula that contains adequate levels of vitamins E and C, beta-carotene, zinc, and copper. Animal studies, observational epidemiological studies, and a few small clinical trials of supplements have suggested that zinc, selenium, lutein, zeaxanthin, beta-carotene, vitamins A, C, and E, and omega-3 fatty acids are associated with decreased risk of AMD and cataracts.

Feeding the Fire!

A diet high in saturated and trans fats is ill advised. You want to avoid highly processed foods devoid of adequate antioxidants.

BETTER VISION MENU PLAN

Day 1

Breakfast (375)
1 cup flaxseed cereal flakes (190)
½ cup stewed apricot (35)
1 cup skim milk (90)
½ cup orange juice (60)
1 cup green tea

Lunch (430)
1 serving *Roasted Vegetable and Sweet Swiss Panini* (250)
(page 333)
6 whole grain crackers (130)
½ cup Concord grapes (50)
1½ cups water with lemon

Midday Snack (300)
1 serving *Chilean Fruit Guacamole* (100) (page 259)
12 fat-free corn chips (120)
½ ounce pistachios (80)
1 cup green tea

Dinner (540)
4 ounces rotisserie chicken (220)
1 cup steamed Brussels sprouts (60)
1 serving *Raw Kale Salad with Lemon-Honey Vinaigrette* (260)
(page 296)
1 cup decaffeinated green tea

Evening Snack (345)
½ cup carrot sticks (25)
1 serving *Sardine Salad/Dip* (320) (page 265)
1 cup decaffeinated green tea

Day 2

Breakfast (530)
1 serving *Soufflé Omelet with Balsamic Strawberries* (160)
(page 345)
1 serving *Pan-Cooked Apples and Pears in Grape Juice* (150)
(page 313)
1 whole grain English muffin (130)
1 cup skim milk (90)

Lunch (440)
1 serving *Blackberry Smoothie* (320) (page 258)
1 serving *Avocado-Fennel Citrus Salad* (120) (page 285)

Midday Snack (370)
2 servings *Kale Balls* (80) (page 262)
1 serving *Rosemary Nuts* (290) (page 269)
1 cup green tea

Dinner (610)
1 serving *Cocoa-Encrusted Salmon with Blueberries* (270)
(page 330)
1 serving *Curried Chickpeas and Kale* (150) (page 370)
1 whole grain roll (100)
1 cup skim milk (90)

Evening Snack (146)
1 serving *Beanie-Greenie Brownies* (110) (page 309)
1 serving *Watermelon Soda* (36) (page 253)

Day 3

Breakfast (415)
1 serving *Chef Wiley's Granola* (290) (page 351)
½ cup stewed apricots (35)
1 cup skim milk (90)
1 cup green tea

Lunch (440)
1 serving *Tropical Fruit and Shrimp Gazpacho* (80) (page 279)
1 serving *Raw Kale Salad with Lemon-Honey Vinaigrette* (260)
(page 296)
1 whole grain roll (100)
1½ cups water with lemon

Midday Snack (260)
1 serving *Strawberry-Papaya Smoothie* (130) (page 255)
1 serving *Spicy Biscotti* (130) (page 311)

Dinner (720)
1 serving *Grilled Chicken Salad with Pomegranate Vinaigrette
and Mango Gelée Garnish* (300) (page 324)
1 small corn on the cob (70)
1 ounce almonds and pistachios (160)
1 whole grain roll (100)
1 cup skim milk (90)

Evening Snack (180)
Polenta Pizza (180) (page 329)
1 cup decaffeinated green tea

Dave's Tips

1. Minimize eye exposure to the sun—wear UV-protective eyewear.
2. Manage diabetes and weight, as these can contribute to poor eyesight.
3. Avoid eating rancid, saturated, and trans fats. They put the pedal to the metal on damage to eyesight.

SECTION TWO

OPTIMAL LIVING RECIPES

BEVERAGES

Watermelon Soda

By Veronica "Roni" Noone
www.greenlitebites.com

SERVINGS: 6

Ingredients
3 cups diced watermelon
1 cup sparkling water
½ orange, sliced thin
4 to 5 large strawberries, hulled and sliced
Crushed ice

Directions
Puree the watermelon in a blender. Pour the puree into a pitcher and mix in the sparkling water. Add the orange and strawberries and let sit until ready to serve. Add ice just before serving.

Nutrition Profile

36 calories, 0 g total fat, 0 g saturated fat, 0 mg cholesterol, 0 mg sodium, 10 g carbs, 1 g fiber, 1 g protein.

Apple-Soy Chai Latte

Courtesy of SOYJOY
www.soyjoy.com

SERVINGS: 2

Ingredients

1 chai tea bag
½ cup boiling water
1 cup vanilla light soy milk
½ cup apple cider
2 tablespoons honey
1 teaspoon ground cinnamon
1 cinnamon stick per serving, for garnish (optional)

Directions

Combine the chai tea bag and boiling water in a coffee mug. Steep for 5 to 10 minutes, until the water turns dark amber. Remove the chai tea bag and discard. Set the steeped chai aside. In a small saucepan, heat the soy milk, apple cider, honey, and ground cinnamon over medium heat, stirring frequently, for about 10 minutes, until frothy. Add the steeped chai to the saucepan and mix. Serve in a large mug. Garnish with the cinnamon stick, if desired.

Nutrition Profile
130 calories, 1 g total fat, 0 g saturated fat, 0 mg cholesterol, 60 mg sodium, 29 g carbs, 1 g fiber, 2 g protein.

Strawberry-Papaya Smoothie

By Veronica "Roni" Noone
www.greenlitebites.com

Roni's Raves—WOW, WOW, WOW! I LOVED THIS! Sorry, I
really had to scream that. It was that good. The papaya texture
is just perfect for this smoothie!

SERVINGS: 1

Ingredients
1 cup diced ripe papaya
¼ cup plain nonfat yogurt
4 large frozen strawberries

Directions
Blend all the ingredients together and serve!

Nutrition Profile
130 calories, 1.5 g total fat, 0.5 g saturated fat, 5 mg cholesterol,
50 mg sodium, 26 g carbs, 5 g fiber, 4 g protein.

Cherry Zinger Smoothie

Developed for the Almond Board of California by
Cynthia Sass, MPH, MA, RD, CSSD
www.almondboard.com

SERVINGS: 1

Ingredients
½ cup vanilla-flavored almond milk
2 tablespoons almond butter
1 cup frozen unsweetened cherries
1 tablespoon honey
1 teaspoon freshly ground coffee beans

Directions
Combine all the ingredients in a blender. Blend until smooth, and serve.

Nutrition Profile
383 calories, 21 g total fat, 2 g saturated fat, 0 mg cholesterol, 221 mg sodium, 49 g carbs, 4.2 g fiber, 7 g protein.

Quick Pumpkin Smoothie

By Veronica "Roni" Noone
www.greenlitebites.com

SERVINGS: 1

Ingredients
½ cup canned pumpkin
½ cup vanilla nonfat yogurt
½ cup vanilla or chocolate soy milk
½ teaspoon pumpkin pie spice
2 to 3 ice cubes
Agave syrup to taste (if added sweetness is desired)

Directions:
Place all the ingredients in a blender and blend until smooth.
Can't get much easier than that!

Nutrition Profile
230 calories, 2 g total fat, 0 g saturated fat, 5 mg cholesterol, 140
mg sodium, 42 g carbs, 5 g fiber, 12 g protein.

Blackberry Smoothie

By Chef Elisa Hunziker
www.cancersurvivorchef.com

SERVINGS: 1

Ingredients
4 ice cubes
¾ cup apple juice
1 cup fresh or frozen blackberries
Juice of 1 orange
1 tablespoon agave syrup
1 tablespoon whey protein
1 tablespoon flaxseeds, ground

Directions
Crush the ice in a blender first, then add the remaining ingredients and blend until smooth.

Nutrition Profile
320 calories, 4.5 g total fat, 0 g saturated fat, 10 mg cholesterol, 25 mg sodium, 67 g carbs, 10 g fiber, 8 g protein.

APPETIZERS

Chilean Fruit Guacamole

Courtesy of the Chilean Avocado Importers Association (CAIA)
www.chileanavocados.org

CAIA's Tip—*You can also use this as a salsa to top burgers,*
fish, pork, or chicken.

SERVINGS: 8

Ingredients
2 Chilean Hass avocados
2 to 3 tablespoons freshly squeezed lime or lemon juice
½ teaspoon salt
Pepper
1 peach, peeled and diced
1 cup halved red or green seedless grapes

¼ cup chopped fresh mint

Dash of Tabasco sauce or cayenne pepper to taste (optional)

Directions

Rinse the avocados and cut in half. With a spoon, remove the pit from each avocado and scoop the flesh into a medium bowl. Add the lime juice, the salt, and pepper to taste, and mash with a fork until the mixture is chunky. (Or spoon into a zip-top plastic bag, seal, and mash with your hands until chunky.) Stir in the peach, grapes, and mint. If desired, add Tabasco sauce or cayenne pepper. Serve with toasted pita triangles or sweet potato chips.

Nutrition Profile

100 calories, 7 g total fat, 1 g saturated fat, 0 mg cholesterol, 150 mg sodium, 8 g carbs, 4 g fiber, 1 g protein.

Royal Blue Cheese—Stuffed Mushrooms

By Sue McCloskey, owner of Ponte Fresco Restaurant in Chicago
www.pontefrescousa.com

Sue's Tip—*I suggest using delicious Royal Blue Cheese from Fair Oaks Farms (www.fofarms.com).*

SERVINGS: 24

Ingredients

24 large mushrooms, cleaned

2 tablespoons extra-virgin olive oil

1 onion, chopped

2 cloves garlic, minced

¼ cup chopped fresh parsley

1 (8-ounce) package nonfat cream cheese, softened and cut into pieces

4 ounces Fair Oaks Farms Royal Blue Cheese, softened and cut into pieces

1 tablespoon freshly squeezed lemon juice

2 tablespoons cream sherry or port wine (optional)

Salt and pepper

Directions

Preheat the oven to 400°F.

Remove the stems from the mushrooms and chop fine. Set the caps aside.

In a large skillet over medium heat, heat the olive oil. Add the chopped mushroom stems, onion, and garlic. Cook, stirring, for 5 to 6 minutes, until the onion is translucent. Reduce the heat to low; add the parsley, cream cheese, blue cheese, lemon juice, and cream sherry or port, if desired. Stir until the cheeses are melted and well blended. Remove from the heat. Season to taste with salt and pepper.

Spoon the cheese mixture into the mushroom caps, filling generously. Place the stuffed mushroom caps on a baking sheet with sides. Bake for 8 to 10 minutes, until the mushrooms are cooked and the cheese is lightly browned. Remove from the heat and place the mushrooms on a large serving plate or platter. Serve immediately.

Nutrition Profile

60 calories, 2 g total fat, 0.5 g saturated fat, 5 mg cholesterol, 130 mg sodium, 6 g carbs, 1 g fiber, 4 g protein.

Kale Balls

By Diana Dyer, MS, RD
www.cancerrd.com

Diana's Tips—*It is important to remove the large tough stems from the kale, but keep the small tender ones. I did use my food processor instead of cutting up the greens to save me time, even though I love to chop, chop, chop with my chef's knife. Serve at a buffet or party, using toothpicks, with some marinara sauce or even some unflavored yogurt for dipping.*

SERVINGS: 28

Ingredients

4 cups water

8 cups chopped kale

3 eggs

1 teaspoon dried Italian herbs

½ teaspoon garlic powder (more if your family really likes garlic, like mine)

½ teaspoon low-sodium tamari

1 to 2 tablespoons extra-virgin olive oil

½ cup freshly grated Parmesan cheese

1 cup dry whole wheat bread crumbs

¼ cup flaxseeds, ground

Directions

Preheat the oven to 350°F.

Place a steamer basket in a large pot. Add the water and bring to a boil. Reduce the heat to medium and cook the chopped kale, covered, for just a few minutes, until the kale turns a bright green color. The kale will reduce to about 4 cups. Drain and set aside to cool.

Lightly beat the eggs in a large bowl, then add all the remaining ingredients (except the kale) and mix together.

Finally add the kale and mix well. Don't be afraid to use your hands at this step to mix everything evenly!

Line a cookie sheet with parchment paper.

Using a teaspoon and your hands, make 28 kale balls, each about 1 inch in diameter, and place on the prepared cookie sheet.

Bake for 15 to 20 minutes, until browned.

Nutrition Profile
40 calories, 1.5 g total fat, 0 g saturated fat, 0 mg cholesterol, 70 mg sodium, 5 g carbs, 1 g fiber, 2 g protein.

Asian Satay Skewers with Black Bean Sauce

Developed for Bush's beans by Connie Guttersen, RD, PhD, nutrition instructor at the Culinary Institute of America and author of The Sonoma Diet *and* The Sonoma Diet Cookbook. *www.vegetablewithmore.com*

Dave's Tip: *I've also substituted turkey, lean pork, tuna, or firm tofu for the chicken with really tasty results!*

SERVINGS: 8

Ingredients

Satay Skewers
1 pound boneless, skinless chicken breast halves, cut into 2 x ½-inch strips

Salt and pepper

1 cup low-sodium teriyaki sauce

1 tablespoon minced peeled fresh ginger

1 tablespoon minced garlic

1 teaspoon light sesame oil

8 (6-inch-long) wooden skewers

1 (12-inch) sheet heavy-duty aluminum foil

Sauce

½ (15-ounce) can Bush's black beans, drained and rinsed

½ (15.8-ounce) can Bush's Great Northern beans, drained and rinsed

1 cup frozen shelled soybeans, thawed

½ cup chopped scallions

1 tablespoon minced peeled fresh ginger

2 tablespoons chopped fresh cilantro

2 tablespoons sugar

2 tablespoons freshly squeezed lime juice

¼ cup low-sodium soy sauce

1 teaspoon minced garlic

1 serrano chile, chopped (optional)

2 teaspoons light sesame oil

Directions

Satay Skewers: Season the chicken strips with salt and pepper. Combine the teriyaki sauce, ginger, garlic, and sesame oil in a medium bowl. Toss the chicken in the marinade. Let marinate in the refrigerator for at least 45 minutes. Weave the chicken strips onto the skewers. Discard the marinade.

To Cook: Preheat the grill to medium-hot. Fold the sheet of heavy-duty foil lengthwise into thirds. Place on the grill along the front edge. Place the satay skewers on the grill, laying the meat ends over the fire and the wood ends on the foil. This will help keep the exposed wood from burning.

Sauce: Combine the beans, soybeans, scallions, ginger, and cilantro in a medium bowl. Mix well. In a small bowl, combine the sugar, lime juice, and soy sauce. Mix until the sugar has dissolved. Add the garlic, chile if desired, and sesame oil. Let sit for 5 minutes. Add the soy sauce mixture to the bean mixture; gently toss to coat.

To Serve: Serve the satay skewers with the bean sauce on the side. Drizzle some of the liquid from the sauce on top of the skewers.

Nutrition Profile
196 calories, 5.5 g total fat, 1 g saturated fat, 32 mg cholesterol, 779 mg sodium, 18 g carbs, 3.5 g fiber, 18.5 g protein.

Sardine Salad/Dip

By Chef Elisa Hunziker
www.cancersurvivorchef.com

SERVINGS: 1

Ingredients
1 (3.75-ounce) can brisling sardines packed in olive oil, drained and cut up
2 tablespoons mayonnaise or Miso Mayo
1 tablespoon finely chopped celery
2 teaspoons chopped fresh flat-leaf parsley
1 teaspoon chopped drained capers
½ teaspoon finely grated lemon zest

1 teaspoon freshly squeezed lemon juice

Salt and pepper

Directions

In a small mixing bowl, combine all the ingredients with a fork. Serve on crackers, as a sandwich spread, or by itself as a wonderful alternative to tuna salad!

Nutrition Profile

320 calories, 4.5 g total fat, 0 g saturated fat, 10 mg cholesterol, 25 mg sodium, 67 g carbs, 10 g fiber, 8 g protein.

Chile-Honey Almond Chicken Kebabs

Developed by Mindy Hermann, MBA, RD, winner of the Almond Board of California's 2009 "Snack Attack" Recipe Contest

www.almondboard.com

Mindy's Tips—*In this recipe, I call for chipotle chiles canned in a spicy tomato sauce known as adobo. You can usually find chipotle chiles in Latin American markets and on the international aisle of many supermarkets. You can also use lean beef, flank steak, shrimp, tuna or salmon, or tempeh or firm tofu in place of the chicken.*

SERVINGS: 10

Ingredients

2 pounds boneless, skinless chicken tenders

2 cups almond milk* or buttermilk

* *Use almond milk if a kosher recipe is desired.*

1 cup almonds, toasted (see page 269)

¾ cup dry whole wheat bread crumbs (from 2 slices whole wheat bread)

1 tablespoon smoked paprika

1 teaspoon salt

½ teaspoon garlic powder

½ teaspoon onion powder

10 (6-inch-long) metal or wood skewers

2 large eggs

1 tablespoon Dijon mustard

Chile-Honey Dipping Sauce (see page 268)

Directions

Cut each tender in half. Place the pieces in a large, shallow dish, add the almond milk, and stir to coat. Cover, and refrigerate for at least 30 minutes or up to 2 hours. Preheat the oven to 400°F.

In a food processor, grind together the almonds, bread crumbs, paprika, salt, garlic powder, and onion powder. Place in a shallow rectangular pan.

Drain the almond milk from the chicken through a colander, discarding the liquid. Thread approximately 4 chicken pieces onto each skewer. In a small bowl, whisk together the eggs and Dijon mustard until smooth. Place in a shallow rectangular pan. Place each chicken skewer in the egg mixture and turn to coat well. Remove from the mixture, allowing the excess to drip off, and place in the almond–bread crumb mixture. Spoon the crumb mixture over each skewer to coat the pieces well.

Remove the skewers from the crumb mixture and place on a baking rack set on top of a rimmed nonstick baking sheet (or spray the baking sheet with cooking spray). Bake for 30 minutes, or until the chicken is fully cooked and the crust is browned.

While the chicken is baking, prepare the dipping sauce. Serve the kebabs warm, with the dipping sauce on the side.

Chile-Honey Dipping Sauce

Ingredients

¾ cup freshly squeezed orange juice

½ cup apple cider vinegar

¼ cup honey

2 tablespoons sugar

1 tablespoon chopped canned chipotle chiles

2 teaspoons freshly squeezed lemon or lime juice

1 tablespoon chili powder

½ teaspoon garlic powder

½ teaspoon onion powder

⅛ teaspoon salt

1½ tablespoons cornstarch (or 2 teaspoons arrowroot) dissolved in ¼ cup water

Directions

Combine all the ingredients except the cornstarch mixture in a small saucepan. Bring to a simmer and cook over low heat, stirring occasionally, for 10 minutes. Add the cornstarch mixture and stir well; simmer over low heat until thickened, about 3 minutes. Keep warm until ready to serve.

Nutrition Profile

Chicken

208 calories, 10.5 g total fat, 1 g saturated fat, 94 mg cholesterol, 668 mg sodium, 6 g carbs, 2 g fiber, 24 g protein.

Sauce

53 calories, 0 g total fat, 0 g saturated fat, 0 mg cholesterol, 49 mg sodium, 13 g carbs, 0 g fiber, 0 g protein.

Rosemary Nuts

*By Chef Elizabeth Wiley, from the Meadowlark Restaurant
in Dayton, Ohio
www.meadowlarkrestaurant.com*

SERVINGS: 28 TO 30 ($\frac{1}{4}$-CUP PORTIONS)

Ingredients

2 pounds assorted unsalted nuts
$\frac{1}{4}$ cup finely chopped fresh rosemary
$\frac{1}{4}$ to $\frac{1}{2}$ teaspoon cayenne pepper
$1\frac{1}{3}$ tablespoons light brown sugar
$1\frac{1}{3}$ tablespoons kosher salt or sea salt
2 tablespoons unsalted butter, melted

Directions

Preheat the oven to 350°F.

Pour the nuts one layer thick onto a baking sheet and bake for 14 minutes or until browned.

Mix the rosemary, cayenne pepper, brown sugar, and salt into the melted butter, and keep warm. The nuts should also be warm when they are added to the butter mixture. Gently reheat either one if they cool before combining.

Pour the butter mixture and warm nuts into a large bowl, and with two wooden spoons, mix thoroughly, coating the nuts with the butter. Let the nuts dry and cool completely before storing them in an airtight container for up to 2 weeks.

Nutrition Profile

290 calories, 16 g total fat, 2.5 g saturated fat, 0 mg cholesterol, 260 mg sodium, 7 g carbs, 3 g fiber, 5 g protein.

"Devils on Horseback"

By Chef Sean O'Brien, from Zinnia Restaurant in San Francisco
www.zinniasf.com

SERVINGS: 12

Ingredients

Apple-Ginger Chutney
5 pounds (about 12 medium) apples, peeled and grated
½ cup sugar
½ cup apple cider vinegar
½ cup minced yellow onion
1 tablespoon grated peeled fresh ginger
1 teaspoon salt
1½ teaspoons minced garlic
½ teaspoon red pepper flakes

Dried Plums
1 cup ruby port
12 California dried plums, pitted
12 almonds
12 thin slices pancetta

Port Reduction
1 cup sugar
½ cup rice wine vinegar
Remaining ruby port/wine (from soaking the dried plums)

12 slices crostini

Directions

Apple-Ginger Chutney: Preheat the oven to 375°F.

Combine all the ingredients in an ovenproof cooking vessel. Cover with parchment and bring to a boil. Transfer to the oven, and bake, covered, for about 45 minutes, until all the juices are concentrated. Stir occasionally. Refrigerate for up to 2 weeks. Yields 6 cups.

Dried Plums: Bring the 1 cup ruby port to a simmer. Remove from the heat, and add the pitted dried plums. Let the plums soak for 10 minutes. Drain, reserving the soaking liquid, and insert 1 whole almond into each plum. Wrap each plum with a slice of pancetta. Sear the plums in a hot pan until the pancetta is slightly crisp.

Port Reduction: Combine all the ingredients and reduce to 1 cup.

To Serve: Place a small amount of the chutney on a crostini, top with a stuffed dried plum, and drizzle with the port reduction. Optional: Serve without the chutney and/or the crostini.

Nutrition Profile

180 calories, 1.5 g total fat, 0 g saturated fat, 0 mg cholesterol, 135 mg sodium, 36 g carbs, 2 g fiber, 3 g protein.

Cheese-and-Fruit Kebabs

Courtesy of Bel Brands USA
www.laughingcow.com

Dave's Tips—*Try these at your next kids' party; the kids love assembling them. The kebabs are also great served with your favorite salad dressing. Try adding cherry tomatoes for added color and taste.*

SERVINGS: 4

Ingredients
6 Mini Babybel light cheese rounds
1 cup diced pineapple
1 cup diced mango
1 cup red seedless grapes
4 (8- to 10-inch) bamboo skewers

Directions
Cut each cheese round in half, making 12 pieces, 3 for each skewer. On each skewer, alternate 3 pieces of the cheese with diced pineapple, diced mango, and grapes until the kebab is complete.

Nutrition Profile
70 calories, 2.5 g total fat, 1 g saturated fat, 10 mg cholesterol, 120 mg sodium, 9 g carbs, 1 g fiber, 5 g protein.

SOUPS AND CHILI

Potato-Corn Chowder

By Sharon Grotto

SERVINGS: 10

Ingredients
2 tablespoons extra-virgin olive oil
2 cups chopped Vidalia onions
1 clove garlic, minced
2 cups chopped carrots
6 cups low-sodium vegetable broth
5 cups diced potatoes
1 (15-ounce) can sweet corn, with liquid
¼ cup chopped fresh parsley
¼ cup chopped fresh dill
½ teaspoon pepper
1½ cups shredded mild Cheddar cheese

Directions

In a large Dutch oven or soup pot, heat the olive oil over medium heat. Add the onions, garlic, and carrots, cover, and simmer over low heat for 20 minutes or until the vegetables are tender. Add the vegetable broth, potatoes, corn, and parsley. Cover and simmer for 30 minutes, or until the potatoes are tender. Remove from the heat. Add the dill and pepper, stir, and cover. Let sit for 5 minutes. Drain the vegetables, reserving the stock, and place in a food processor; process until creamy or until the desired texture is achieved. Return the pureed vegetables to the stock and simmer over low heat. Gradually add the cheese while stirring. Serve.

Nutrition Profile

220 calories, 9 g total fat, 4 g saturated fat, 15 mg cholesterol, 340 mg sodium, 29 g carbs, 4 g fiber, 7 g protein.

Garlic Pipérade Soup

By Chef Cheryl Bell, MS, RD, LDN, CHE

SERVINGS: 6

Ingredients

1 tablespoon extra-virgin olive oil
2 cups chopped onions
1 cup diced red bell pepper
20 cloves garlic, sliced
3 cups diced peeled ripe tomatoes
2 cups low-sodium vegetable broth
3 to 4 slices whole wheat bread, cubed

Freshly ground black pepper, for garnish
Freshly grated Parmesan cheese, for garnish

Directions
In a 2-quart saucepan, heat the oil over medium heat. Add the
onions and bell pepper. Cook until the vegetables are softened,
about 5 minutes. Add the garlic and tomatoes. Reduce the heat,
cover the pan, and simmer for 30 minutes. Add the broth and
bring to a boil. Remove from the heat, and add the bread cubes.
Garnish each serving with black pepper and cheese.

Nutrition Profile
150 calories, 3 g total fat, 0 g saturated fat, 0 mg cholesterol, 360
mg sodium, 26 g carbs, 4 g fiber, 4 g protein.

Gazpacho

By Chef Carrie Walters, from Dorothy Lane Market in Dayton, Ohio
www.dorothylane.com

SERVINGS: 8

Ingredients
1 clove garlic, minced
¼ cup extra-virgin olive oil
1 cup torn-up firm whole wheat bread
2 pounds ripe tomatoes, quartered and cored
1 green bell pepper, chopped
8 scallions, chopped
1 large cucumber, peeled and chopped
2 tablespoons white wine vinegar

1 tablespoon freshly squeezed lemon juice

¼ teaspoon dried tarragon

Salt and pepper

¼ to ½ teaspoon Tabasco sauce

½ teaspoon sugar

2 cups low-sodium chicken broth

1½ cups tomato juice

¼ cup white wine

Garnishes

½ cup diced tomato

½ cup diced peeled cucumber

½ cup diced green bell pepper

Garlic croutons

Crème fraîche or sour cream

Directions

Sauté the garlic in the oil until soft and fragrant, 1 to 2 minutes. Set aside.

Puree the bread, tomatoes, and garlic oil in a food processor. Add the bell pepper, scallions, cucumber, vinegar, lemon juice, tarragon, salt and pepper to taste, Tabasco, and sugar. Puree. Strain if you wish. Stir in the chicken broth, tomato juice, and white wine. Adjust the seasonings, adding more Tabasco if desired.

Cover and refrigerate for at least several hours or up to 2 days. To serve, place the soup in large, shallow bowls and garnish. (Garnishes should be served in bowls at the table for diners to choose.)

Nutrition Profile

130 calories, 7 g total fat, 1 g saturated fat, 0 mg cholesterol, 310 mg sodium, 14 g carbs, 2 g fiber, 3 g protein.

Winter Squash Soup with Roasted Seeds

By Veronica "Roni" Noone
www.greenlitebites.com

Roni's Raves—*This is my attempt to re-create the Autumn Butternut Squash Soup from the Dogwood Gourmet (www .dogwoodbaltimore.com), an awesome Baltimore catering company focusing on local farms and businesses for their menu items. The seeds add a great texture and the soup has that wonderful creamy squash texture without adding any extra cream. What a great way to start a meal.*

SERVINGS: 8

Ingredients
1 small acorn squash
1 butternut squash
1 red apple, peeled
Kosher salt
1 teaspoon coriander seeds
1 teaspoon ground cumin
⅛ teaspoon pepper
½ teaspoon ground ginger
⅛ teaspoon ground cloves
¼ teaspoon ground cinnamon
2 cups of your favorite low-sodium vegetable or chicken broth
2 bay leaves
Dried parsley, for garnish

Directions
Preheat the oven to 350°F.

Cut both squashes in half, scraping out and saving the seeds. Core the apple. Line a cookie sheet with aluminum foil and spray with cooking spray. Lay the squash, flesh side down, on the cookie sheet; place the apple on the same cookie sheet; and bake for 45 minutes to 1 hour or until individually tender. Remove and let cool for a few minutes.

While the squash is baking, clean the pulp from the seeds, rinse them, and allow them to dry on a paper towel.

While the squash and apple are cooling, line another cookie sheet with foil and spray with cooking spray. Lay the squash seeds out and sprinkle with kosher salt. Bake for 10 to 15 minutes, until toasted.

While the squash seeds are toasting, add the coriander seeds, cumin, pepper, ginger, cloves, cinnamon, squash, apple, and broth to a blender. You are going to have to do about three "batches," as it's a lot of soup. Start with all the spices and half the acorn and butternut squash, and keep adding broth until all is well blended. Then pour about half out into a pot over low heat, add more squash, and blend with additional broth. Keep repeating this process until you are out of squash and broth. When finished, mix well in the pot. Add the bay leaves. Continue to simmer for at least 10 to 15 minutes until ready to serve.

Remove the bay leaves. Place 2 ladlefuls, about 1 cup, in each bowl and sprinkle with about 1 tablespoon of the toasted seeds and a pinch of dried parsley.

Nutrition Profile
70 calories, 0 g total fat, 0 g saturated fat, 0 mg cholesterol, 120 mg sodium, 16 g carbs, 3 g fiber, 1 g protein.

Tropical Fruit and Shrimp Gazpacho

By Chef Owen Tilley, Corporate Executive Chef and Director of Culinary, High Liner Foods, Nova Scotia
www.highlinerfoods.com

SERVINGS: 12

Ingredients
8 cups low-sodium V8 juice
½ cup passion fruit nectar
½ cup diced mango
½ cup diced peeled cucumber
¼ cup diced green bell pepper
¼ cup diced tomato
¼ cup chopped fresh cilantro
¼ cup diced papaya
¼ cup freshly squeezed lime juice
¼ cup diced red onion
1 tablespoon Tabasco sauce
1 tablespoon cumin seeds, toasted in a dry skillet and ground
Salt

Garnishes
1 cup chopped cooked shrimp
12 lime wheels
12 sprigs fresh cilantro

Directions
Combine all the ingredients (except the garnishes) in an airtight container and refrigerate. Allow 24 hours for the flavors to develop. Serve in a large, shallow bowl, preferably chilled. Garnish

with the chopped cooked shrimp, lime wheels, and cilantro sprigs.

Nutrition Profile
80 calories, 0 g total fat, 0 g saturated fat, 40 mg cholesterol, 170 mg sodium, 11 g carbs, 2 g fiber, 6 g protein.

Curried Chicken-Banana-Yam Soup

By Chef Gail Roloff, from CHOW restaurant in Elmhurst, Illinois
www.chowtogo.com

SERVINGS: 8

Ingredients
2 teaspoons peanut oil
2 teaspoons extra-virgin olive oil
1½ pounds Amish or organic chicken pieces (legs, thighs, and breasts)
1 small leek, sliced and rinsed
1 small yellow onion, chopped
1 clove garlic, peeled
½ jalapeño pepper
1 tablespoon minced peeled fresh ginger
1 tablespoon mild curry powder
⅛ teaspoon cayenne pepper
1 (14.5-ounce) can diced tomatoes
½ cup shredded unsweetened dried coconut
4 cups low-sodium chicken broth
1 yam or sweet potato, peeled and cut into large dice

Approximately 2 medium bananas, peeled and cut into large
pieces (1 cup)
4 ounces fresh cilantro, chopped
2 tablespoons honey
Sea salt and pepper to taste

Directions

In a heavy-bottomed pot or Dutch oven, heat the oils over
medium heat. Sear the chicken pieces in the hot oils until
browned on each side. Remove from the pot and set aside. Add
the leek and onion. Sweat for a minute; then add the garlic,
jalapeño, and ginger and cook for another minute. Add the curry
powder and cayenne pepper. Stir and toast the spices for a mo-
ment and then add the tomatoes, coconut, chicken stock, and
browned chicken pieces. Stir to combine and bring this mixture
to a rapid boil. Reduce heat. Stir in the yam and reduce heat to
simmer. Cook for 30 to 40 minutes, until the chicken is fully
cooked and falling off the bones and the yam is tender. Pull the
soup off the heat and remove the chicken pieces; let them cool a
bit and then shred the meat. Discard the skin and bones. Stir
the chicken meat, bananas, cilantro, and honey into the pot. Put
back on the heat and simmer for 8 to 10 more minutes. Season
with sea salt and pepper.

Nutrition Profile

280 calories, 15 g total fat, 5 g saturated fat, 65 mg cholesterol,
450 mg sodium, 13 g carbs, 3 g fiber, 23 g protein.

Winter White Bean Chili
(Slow-Cooker Recipe)

Developed for Bush's beans by Connie Guttersen, RD, PhD, nutrition instructor at the Culinary Institute of America and author of The Sonoma Diet *and* The Sonoma Diet Cookbook
www.vegetablewithmore.com

SERVINGS: 9

Ingredients
1 tablespoon extra-virgin olive oil
1 cup chopped onions
1 cup chopped celery
2 tablespoons minced garlic
1 cup chopped carrots
1 pound boneless, skinless chicken breast halves
2 cups chopped zucchini
½ cup brown rice (not instant)
2½ cups low-sodium chicken broth
8 ounces canned mild Mexican green chiles
¼ teaspoon ground cumin
2 (15.8-ounce) cans Bush's Great Northern beans, with liquid
1 tablespoon chopped fresh oregano
1 tablespoon chopped fresh parsley
Salt and pepper
Shredded Colby–Monterey Jack cheese
Salsa verde

Directions
Heat the olive oil over medium heat in a medium skillet. Add the onions, celery, and garlic. Cook, stirring, until the garlic is

aromatic, approximately 5 minutes. Place the carrots in the bottom of a 4-quart slow cooker. Top with the chicken and sautéed onion mixture. Add the zucchini, rice, chicken broth, chiles, cumin, and beans. Cook on high for 4 hours, or until the vegetables and chicken are tender. Remove the chicken breasts and shred them. Mix the chicken back in and add the oregano and parsley. Cook for 5 minutes more. Season with salt and pepper. Serve with the desired amounts of cheese and salsa verde on top.

Nutrition Profile (without the cheese and salsa verde)
257 calories, 6 g total fat, 2 g saturated fat, 31 mg cholesterol, 851 mg sodium, 30 g carbs, 7.5 g fiber, 20 g protein.

SALADS

Avocado-Fennel Citrus Salad

Courtesy of the Chilean Avocado Importers Association (CAIA)
www.chileanavocados.org

SERVINGS: 8

Ingredients
1 grapefruit
2 oranges
2 Chilean Hass avocados
1 to 2 tablespoons honey
1 tablespoon fresh lime or lemon juice
½ teaspoon salt
1 fennel bulb, trimmed and sliced very thin (reserve fronds for garnish)

Directions

Working over a large bowl to catch the juices and the fruit, peel and section the grapefruit and oranges. Rinse the avocados, cut in half, and spoon out the pits. Remove the peel. Cut the flesh into slices or chunks, reserving a few slices for garnish. Add to the grapefruit mixture and toss gently to coat with the juices. Drain the juices off into a small bowl; stir in the honey, lime juice, and salt. Add the fennel slices and the juice mixture to the fruit mixture and toss gently to combine. Garnish with fennel fronds and slices of avocado.

Nutrition Profile

120 calories, 5 g total fat, 0.5 g saturated fat, 0 mg cholesterol, 160 mg sodium, 19 g carbs, 5 g fiber, 2 g protein.

Nuts and Berry Fruit Salad

By Debbie Reynolds, Jeff Mahlmann, Ellen Burbage,
Jan Cappuccio, James Hewson, and Pat Horvath
Courtesy of Lockheed Martin
www.lockheedmartin.com

Dave's Tip—*This salad was created during a mock "Iron Chef" exercise I conducted, where competitive groups had to come up with a delicious and healthy dish in thirty minutes, using any of the 101 foods available to them. Hope you enjoy this winning salad!*

SERVINGS: 2

Ingredients

3 cups cut-up romaine lettuce

1 tablespoon freshly squeezed lime juice

$\frac{1}{4}$ cup dried cranberries

$\frac{1}{4}$ cup walnut halves

$\frac{1}{2}$ cup sliced green apple

$\frac{1}{2}$ cup sliced button mushrooms

Salt and pepper

$\frac{1}{4}$ cup balsamic vinegar–and–olive oil dressing of your choice, for garnish

$\frac{1}{2}$ avocado, sliced, for garnish

$\frac{1}{8}$ cup sliced Kalamata olives, for garnish

Directions

Toss all the ingredients except the dressing and olive and avocado slices in a bowl and mix well. Garnish with the dressing and the avocado and olive slices.

Nutrition Profile

350 calories, 26 g total fat, 2.5 g saturated fat, 0 mg cholesterol, 530 mg sodium, 29 g carbs, 6 g fiber, 5 g protein.

Barley Salad with Edamame

Courtesy of SOYJOY

www.soyjoy.com

SOYJOY Tip—*To make this light and tasty dish as easy as possible, look for frozen shelled edamame and packages of preshredded carrots and cabbage.*

SERVINGS: 8

Ingredients:
⅔ cup pearl barley
2 cups frozen shelled edamame
1 cup shredded carrots
3 cups shredded cabbage
½ cup chopped scallions
Low-fat Asian dressing of your choice
Salt and pepper

Directions
Prepare the barley and edamame according to the package instructions. In a medium bowl, toss all the ingredients until the dressing is evenly distributed. Serve warm or cold.

Nutrition Profile
160 calories, 3 g total fat, 0 g saturated fat, 0 mg cholesterol, 190 mg sodium, 25 g carbs, 6 g fiber, 7 g protein.

Mango-Tango Tilapia Salad

By Chef Owen Tilley, Corporate Executive Chef and Director of Culinary, High Liner Foods, Nova Scotia
www.highlinerfoods.com

SERVINGS: 4

Ingredients
4 pieces High Liner Sea Cuisine tortilla-crusted tilapia (about 4 ounces each; can substitute 3- to 4-ounce tilapia fillets)

1 cup diced mango
½ cup fresh or canned diced pineapple chunks
¼ cup sliced roasted red bell pepper
¼ cup julienned red onion
4 tomatoes, quartered
¼ cup sliced pickled jarred red peppers
¼ cup chopped fresh oregano
2 heads romaine lettuce, chopped
¾ cup Catalina dressing

Garnish
2 tablespoons sunflower seed kernels, toasted in a dry skillet
1 lime, quartered

Directions
Cook the tortilla-crusted tilapia as directed, or bake the tilapia fillets in a 400°F oven for 8 to 10 minutes, or until done. While the tilapia cooks, toss all the remaining ingredients, except the dressing, in a large bowl. Dress with the Catalina dressing. Divide among four bowls and place one piece of cooked tilapia atop each salad. Garnish with the sunflower seed kernels and a lime wedge.

Nutrition Profile
270 calories, 4 g total fat, 1 g saturated fat, 55 mg cholesterol, 660 mg sodium, 32 g carbs, 5 g fiber, 26 g protein.

Bean-Corn Salad

By Veronica "Roni" Noone
www.greenlitebites.com

Roni's Tips—*I created this simple no-cook, multipurpose, filling "salsa salad." (Can you tell I had no idea what to call it?) It's great as a topping for sandwiches, on a more traditional salad, or as a filling for lettuce wraps. Yum! Yum! Yum!*

SERVINGS: 6

Ingredients

1 (15-ounce) can red kidney beans, drained and rinsed
1 (8-ounce) can sweet corn, drained and rinsed
2 to 3 slices red onion, cut into small dice
1 tablespoon honey
1 tablespoon freshly squeezed lime juice
1 tablespoon chopped fresh cilantro
1 teaspoon chili powder
½ teaspoon ground cumin
1 teaspoon Tabasco sauce (or to taste)

Directions

Mix all the ingredients and let the salad sit for at least 20 minutes. That's it! The longer it sits, the more the flavors merge.

Nutrition Profile

120 calories, 1 g total fat, 0 g saturated fat, 0 mg cholesterol, 150 mg sodium, 22 g carbs, 5 g fiber, 6 g protein.

Sicilian Broccoli Salad

*By Chef Elizabeth Wiley, from the Meadowlark Restaurant
in Dayton, Ohio*
www.meadowlarkrestaurant.com

Chef Wiley's Tip—*Sicilians might add anchovies and/or
raisins to this dish!*

SERVINGS: 6

Ingredients
Kosher salt
1 bunch broccoli
½ cup extra-virgin olive oil
3 to 4 cloves garlic, minced
Zest of 1 lemon
Zest of ½ orange
Salt and pepper

Directions
Bring a good-sized pot of water with 2 tablespoons of kosher salt
to a boil. Meanwhile, trim the broccoli to medium florets. Add the
broccoli to the boiling water and cook for 3 to 4 minutes, until
brilliantly green. Drain in a colander and cool with cold water.
When cool enough to handle, gently squeeze the florets to get rid
of the excess water. Put into a dry bowl.

Put the ½ cup olive oil in a small saucepan. Add the minced
garlic, turn the heat to medium, and cook, stirring, until the garlic begins to sizzle. When the garlic begins to color, remove the
pan from the heat and let the garlic steep in the oil.

Sprinkle the lemon and orange zest over the broccoli and stir to avoid clumping. Strain the garlic oil, discarding the garlic, and add to the broccoli by the spoonful until the salad is dressed the way you want it. Season with salt and pepper. Mix thoroughly and enjoy!

Dave's Tip—*As Chef Wiley says, "Add the garlic oil by the spoonful until the salad is dressed the way you want it." You may find that you don't need all of the ½ cup of garlic oil on your salad. If that is the case, please consider the calorie and fat content on the high side in the nutrition profile below.*

Nutrition Profile
200 calories, 19 g total fat, 2.5 g saturated fat, 0 mg cholesterol, 35 mg sodium, 7 g carbs, 3 g fiber, 3 g protein.

Grilled Vidalia Onion and Peach Salad

By Chef Jon Ashton, courtesy of the Vidalia Onion Committee
www.vidaliaonion.org

Chef Ashton's Rave—*The sweetness of Vidalia onions and peaches is best showcased in recipes that are not overloaded with other ingredients. This salad, featuring grilled Vidalia onions, is simple, but sure to deliver a unique burst of flavor.*

SERVINGS: 2

Ingredients

Salad
1 cup baby lettuce leaves

1 Vidalia onion, sliced into ½-inch rings
Extra-virgin olive oil, for brushing
Salt and pepper
1 peach, peeled, halved, and pitted

Dressing
1 teaspoon Dijon mustard
1 tablespoon white wine vinegar
2 tablespoons extra-virgin olive oil
Salt and pepper

¼ cup crumbled goat cheese, for garnish

Directions
Salad: Preheat the grill to medium-hot. Place the baby lettuce leaves in a large bowl. Brush the sliced Vidalia onion with olive oil; season with salt and pepper. Grill the onion slices and peach halves until tender, about 4 minutes per side. Thinly slice the peach halves.
Dressing: Simply whisk together all the ingredients in a small bowl.
To serve: Toss together the baby lettuce leaves and the freshly grilled Vidalia onions and sliced peach. Drizzle with the dressing and sprinkle the goat cheese on top. Serve immediately.

Nutrition Profile
270 calories, 21 g total fat, 6 g saturated fat, 15 mg cholesterol, 190 mg sodium, 17 g carbs, 3 g fiber, 6 g protein.

Watermelon and Feta Salad

By Chef Carrie Walters, from Dorothy Lane Market in Dayton, Ohio
www.dorothylane.com

Chef Walter's Tip—*This salad is best if eaten the day that it is made.*

SERVINGS: 2

Ingredients
1 (9-pound) seedless watermelon (9 pounds will yield about 4½ pounds of usable fruit)
1 yellow onion
1 cup pitted Kalamata olives
8 ounces feta cheese
3 tablespoons chopped fresh mint
½ cup extra-virgin olive oil
¼ cup red wine vinegar
1 teaspoon sea salt
½ teaspoon pepper

Directions
Cut the rind off the watermelon. Cut the watermelon into bite-sized pieces. Place in a large bowl. Cut the onion in half from the root end to the stem end. Cut lengthwise again into thin slices. Cut once more in half so you have about 1-inch-long julienne. Cut the Kalamatas lengthwise in half. Cut the feta into bite-sized pieces. Add the onion, olives, feta, and mint to the bowl with the watermelon. In a separate small bowl, whisk the oil, vinegar, salt, and pepper together and pour over the salad, tossing lightly.

Nutrition Profile
270 calories, 19 g total fat, 5 g saturated fat, 10 mg cholesterol, 380 mg sodium, 28 g carbs, 2 g fiber, 6 g protein.

Warm Goat Cheese Salad with Hazelnuts and Raspberries

By Chef Carrie Walters, from Dorothy Lane Market in Dayton, Ohio
www.dorothylane.com

SERVINGS: 6

Ingredients

Salad
1 small log goat cheese
1 cup dry whole wheat bread crumbs
Olive oil cooking spray
8 ounces mesclun or baby lettuce

Raspberry-Mustard Vinaigrette
1 clove garlic, minced
2 tablespoons good-quality whole seed mustard
1 tablespoon raspberry vinegar
1 tablespoon raspberry preserves
6 tablespoons extra-virgin olive oil
Salt and pepper

Garnishes
½ cup hazelnuts, toasted (see page 359) and skinned
1 cup fresh raspberries

Directions

Salad: Preheat the oven to 350°F. Cut the goat cheese into slices about 1 inch thick. Lightly press the cheese slices into the bread crumbs. Mist lightly with oil. Place on a parchment-lined baking sheet. Bake for about 10 minutes or until golden brown. While the cheese is baking, line salad plates with the greens.

Dressing: Combine the minced garlic with the mustard; add the vinegar and preserves. Whisk in the oil until creamy, and season with salt and pepper.

To serve: Place a warm goat cheese medallion on top of the greens. Scatter with the nuts and fresh raspberries. Drizzle with the dressing. Serve.

Nutrition Profile

390 calories, 29 g total fat, 8 g saturated fat, 20 mg cholesterol, 420 mg sodium, 24 g carbs, 2 g fiber, 11 g protein.

Raw Kale Salad with Lemon-Honey Vinaigrette

By Chef Robin Kirby, from CHOW restaurant in Elmhurst, Illinois
www.chowtogo.com

SERVINGS: 6 TO 8

Ingredients

Salad
2 bunches kale, stems and ribs removed, torn into bite-sized pieces
½ cup pomegranate seeds (can substitute dried cranberries)

½ cup diced red onion
½ cup sunflower seeds, shelled

Lemon-Honey Vinaigrette
3 tablespoons freshly squeezed lemon juice
½ cup extra-virgin olive oil
⅛ teaspoon ground cinnamon
2 tablespoons honey
Sea salt and pepper

Directions:
Combine the four salad ingredients in a large bowl. Whisk together the vinaigrette ingredients and toss with the salad. Refrigerate the salad for at least 1 hour prior to serving, to allow the flavors to develop. Serve.

Nutrition Profile
260 calories, 19 g total fat, 2.5 saturated fat, 0 mg cholesterol, 75 mg sodium, 19 g carbs, 2 g fiber, 5 g protein.

Sweet Vidalia Onion Slaw with Fennel, Cucumber, and Champagne-Orange Dressing

By Chef Brian Stapleton, courtesy of the Vidalia Onion Committee
www.vidaliaonion.org

Chef Stapleton's Tips—*This is a nice light salad, perfect for holiday parties or served as a light accompaniment for a casual dinner.*

SERVINGS: 4

Ingredients

Dressing
1 shallot, finely chopped
1 clove garlic, finely chopped
Grated zest and juice of 1 orange
6 tablespoons extra-virgin olive oil
2 tablespoons champagne vinegar
Salt and pepper

Salad
$\frac{1}{2}$ fennel bulb, trimmed and sliced thin
$\frac{1}{2}$ cucumber, peeled, seeded, and sliced thin
1 Vidalia onion, sliced thin
$\frac{1}{2}$ bunch fresh chives, chopped

Directions
Dressing: Using a mixing bowl, combine the shallot, garlic, orange zest, orange juice, olive oil, and vinegar; blend or mix thoroughly. Season to taste with salt and pepper. (The dressing can be made 1 day in advance.)
Salad: One hour before the slaw will be served, using a mixing bowl, combine the fennel, cucumber, Vidalia onion, chives, and dressing. Toss, and adjust the seasonings.

Nutrition Profile
250 calories, 21 g total fat, 3 g saturated fat, 0 mg cholesterol, 20 mg sodium, 15 g carbs, 3 g fiber, 2 g protein.

DRESSINGS AND SAUCES

Raspberry Salsa

Courtesy of the Washington Red Raspberry Commission
www.raspberryinfo.com

SERVINGS: 12

Dave's Tips—*A little sweet, a little sour, a little spicy, and a little crunchy, this salsa is a perfect accompaniment to pork, chicken, fish, or beef. It's also great over sliced fresh fruit or as a complement to a cheese tray. If you prepare and refrigerate the salsa in advance, the jicama and apple will turn a pretty pink from the raspberries.*

Ingredients
2 cups diced peeled jicama
1 Pink Lady or other tart-sweet apple, cored and diced

⅓ cup raspberry vinegar

1 jalapeño pepper, seeded and finely chopped

3 scallions, sliced

1 tablespoon grated peeled fresh ginger

1 (12-ounce) bag frozen Washington raspberries, thawed

Directions

In a large bowl, toss the jicama and apple with the vinegar. Add all the remaining ingredients and toss to blend. Serve at once, or cover and refrigerate until ready to serve.

Nutrition Profile

30 calories, 0 g total fat, 0 g saturated fat, 0 mg cholesterol, 3 mg sodium, 8 g carbs, 3 g fiber, 1 g protein.

Avocado Chimichurri

Courtesy of the Chilean Avocado Importers Association (CAIA)
www.chileanavocados.org

CAIA's Raves—*Chimichurri, a South American condiment, is traditionally a combination of olive oil, vinegar, parsley, garlic, salt, and peppers. It has become the trendy sauce on many restaurant menus, and home cooks are discovering how much zip it can add to steaks, seafood, and poultry, and how fantastic it is as a sandwich spread. This Latin American–fusion version features Chilean avocados, which add rich flavor and a creamy texture.*

SERVINGS: 4 (AS A SAUCE)

Ingredients

1 large Chilean Hass avocado

$\frac{1}{4}$ cup apple cider or other vinegar

1 cup finely chopped fresh curly- or flat-leaf parsley, cilantro, or basil

1 to 2 cloves garlic, minced

$\frac{1}{2}$ teaspoon salt

1 jalapeño pepper, seeded and finely chopped, or several dashes of Tabasco sauce

Directions

Rinse the avocado, cut it in half, and spoon out the pit. Scoop the flesh into a medium bowl. Mash with a fork. Stir in all the remaining ingredients.

Nutrition Profile

80 calories, 6 g total fat, 1 g saturated fat, 0 mg cholesterol, 300 mg sodium, 7 g carbs, 3 g fiber, 1 g protein.

Indian-Style Green Sauce

By Chef Elizabeth Wiley, from the Meadowlark Restaurant
in Dayton, Ohio
www.meadowlarkrestaurant.com

SERVINGS: 15

Ingredients

1 cup almonds, toasted (see page 359)

1 bunch fresh cilantro

1 bunch fresh parsley (preferably flat-leaf)

1 teaspoon minced garlic
¼ cup freshly squeezed lemon juice
¼ cup honey
½ teaspoon chili garlic sauce
1 teaspoon salt
⅛ teaspoon pepper
1 tablespoon sesame oil
1 cup canola oil
⅔ cup water

Directions
In a food processor, grind the toasted almonds.

Clean the cilantro and parsley and discard the bottom 2 to 3 inches of stem, then chop the bunches crosswise into 2-inch pieces. Add to the almonds in the processor along with all the remaining ingredients except the sesame oil, canola oil, and water. Process finely. Once the sauce is smooth, with the machine running, add the oils and water. Drizzle in more water if too thick. Taste for seasoning.

Nutrition Profile
200 calories, 21 g total fat, 1.5 g saturated fat, 0 mg cholesterol, 160 mg sodium, 3 g carbs, 1 g fiber, 2 g protein.

Fruit and Walnut Jam Conserve

Courtesy of Welch's
www.welchs.com

Welch's Tips—*Top pancakes or oatmeal at breakfast, add to chicken salad, or for an elegant and festive treat, serve this*

*chunky jam conserve with blue cheese and thinly sliced bread
or crackers.*

SERVINGS: 32

Ingredients
½ cup coarsely chopped walnuts
¼ cup Welch's white grape juice
¼ cup Welch's purple grape juice
1 large Granny Smith or Golden Delicious apple, cored and
finely diced
1 large firm pear (Bosc or Anjou or Bartlett), cored and finely diced
1 small orange, peeled and finely chopped
1 tablespoon light brown sugar
½ cup Welch's mixed dried fruits
1 shallot, minced
½ teaspoon ground cinnamon
½ teaspoon ground ginger, or 1 teaspoon grated peeled fresh
ginger

Directions
Toast the walnuts in a dry skillet on the stovetop or in the oven
(see page 359).

In a heavy saucepan over medium-high heat, combine the
juices, apple, pear, orange, brown sugar, dried fruits, shallot, cinnamon, and ginger. Bring to a boil and cook, stirring frequently,
until the apple and pear are tender, about 20 minutes.

Stir in the toasted walnuts. Transfer to a small bowl and let
cool. Serve at room temperature.

Nutrition Profile
30 calories, 1 g total fat, 0 g saturated fat, 0 mg cholesterol, 0 mg
sodium, 5 g carbs, 1 g fiber, 1 g protein.

Super Fruit Relish

Courtesy of the Cherry Marketing Institute
www.choosecherries.com

Dave's Tip—*Serve this relish with roasted turkey, duck, chicken, or pork. The relish will keep, covered and chilled, for up to 2 weeks.*

SERVINGS: 16

Ingredients
1½ cups tart cherry juice
12 ounces fresh or frozen cranberries
1½ cups dried cherries
½ teaspoon ground cinnamon
¼ teaspoon ground cloves or ginger
10 ounces currant jelly

Directions
Combine the cherry juice and cranberries in a large saucepan; bring to a boil over high heat. Stir in the dried cherries, cinnamon, and cloves. Reduce the heat; simmer, uncovered, stirring occasionally, for 8 minutes, or until the mixture thickens. Stir in the jelly; simmer, uncovered, stirring occasionally, for 2 minutes. Transfer to a bowl. Refrigerate for at least 4 hours before serving.

Nutrition Profile
110 calories, 0 g total fat, 0 g saturated fat, 0 mg cholesterol, 2 mg sodium, 27 g carbs, 2 g fiber, 1 g protein.

Yogurt Sauce

By Chef Elizabeth Wiley, from the Meadowlark Restaurant
in Dayton, Ohio
www.meadowlarkrestaurant.com

SERVINGS: 8

Ingredients
1 cup plain nonfat yogurt
1½ teaspoons sherry vinegar
2½ teaspoons extra-virgin olive oil
¼ teaspoon salt
¼ teaspoon pepper

Directions
Whisk all the ingredients together thoroughly and serve over salad, with pita wedges. . . . Be creative!

Nutrition Profile
30 calories, 2.5 g total fat, 1 g saturated fat, 0 mg cholesterol, 85 mg sodium, 1 g carbs, 0 g fiber, 1 g protein.

Creamy Avocado Dressing

Courtesy of the Chilean Avocado Importers Association (CAIA)
www.chileanavocados.org

CAIA's Tips—*Thick, creamy, and beautifully green, this easy blend makes a magnificent dressing as well as adding avocado's nutty flavor to a salad. You could replace the basil with parsley, oregano, or even dill for a variation. In addition to topping salad greens, try the dressing on burgers or steaks, over fish or poultry, or as a dip for fresh vegetable crudités.*

SERVINGS: 16

Ingredients
1 Chilean Hass avocado
¾ cup buttermilk
2 scallions, chopped
2 tablespoons packed fresh basil leaves
2 tablespoons white wine vinegar or raspberry vinegar
¼ teaspoon salt

Directions
Rinse the avocado and cut in half. Spoon out the pit. Scoop the flesh into a blender container or food processor bowl. Add all the remaining ingredients and blend until very smooth, about 30 seconds. Can be stored in a tightly covered container in the refrigerator for up to 3 days.

Nutrition Profile
20 calories, 1.5 g total fat, 0 g saturated fat, 0 mg cholesterol, 50 mg sodium, 1 g carbs, 1 g fiber, 1 g protein.

DESSERTS

Poached Pears

By Chef Cheryl Bell, MS, RD, LDN, CHE

SERVINGS: 12

Ingredients
3 cups red wine
½ cup agave syrup
1 cinnamon stick
1 whole clove
¼ teaspoon grated lemon zest
2 black peppercorns
1 bay leaf
6 pears, peeled and cored from the bottom, leaving the stems intact

Directions

In a saucepan, combine all the ingredients except the pears. Bring to a boil while stirring well. Simmer for 5 minutes, then slip the pears into the syrup. Cover and simmer until the pears are tender, about 25 minutes. Using a slotted spoon, remove the pears and place in a serving bowl. Cover and refrigerate.

Pour the syrup through a fine-mesh strainer to remove the solids. Discard the solids. In a saucepan, reduce the syrup over high heat until it is thick enough to coat the back of a spoon, then allow the syrup to cool. Pour over the pears and refrigerate.

Nutrition Profile

165 calories, 0 g total fat, 0 g saturated fat, 0 mg cholesterol, 3 mg sodium, 28 g carbs, 1 g fiber, 0 g protein.

Christine's Baked Custard

By Christine Gerbstadt, MD, RD
www.nutronicsinc.com

Dr. Gerbstadt's Tips—*This recipe may be made with skim milk to reduce the fat per serving to negligible, and with a low-calorie sweetener to reduce the carbohydrates. Taste and / or texture may be altered.*

SERVINGS: 4

Ingredients

2 large eggs

2 cups 2% milk

3 tablespoons honey

½ teaspoon vanilla extract
Dash of ground nutmeg
Dash of ground cinnamon

Directions
Preheat the oven to 325°F. Place a pan in the oven large enough to hold a casserole and fill it with enough hot water to go halfway up the sides of the dish.

Whip the eggs in a bowl and add the milk, honey, vanilla, and spices. Pour into a casserole and place in the oven inside the water bath. Bake for 50 to 60 minutes, until the center is set. Serve warm or chilled.

Nutrition Profile
140 calories, 3.5 g total fat, 1.5 g saturated fat, 115 mg cholesterol, 100 mg sodium, 20 g carbs, 0 g fiber, 8 g protein.

Beanie-Greenie Brownies

By Deb Schiff, author of the blog Altered Plates
alteredplates.blogspot.com

Deb's Tips—*These fudgy brownies hide all kinds of healthy things, including beans! It doesn't matter if they are white, pinto, black. . . . You won't taste them at all. Trust me. I made them carob, but they could be made chocolate just as easily. Just remember to use high-quality unsweetened dark chocolate and cocoa instead.*

Dave's Note: *The original recipe called for coconut flour, but I had a hard time finding it. Deb says that it can be purchased* *online if you can't find it at your local grocery or health food store.*

SERVINGS: 48

Ingredients

1½ cups unsweetened carob chips

3 tablespoons Earth Balance buttery spread, plus more for the pan

¼ cup tahini

1 cup whipped avocado (easily done in a blender or with an immersion blender)

¾ cup pureed cooked beans

1 teaspoon baking powder

1 teaspoon baking soda

1 cup whole wheat pastry flour

¼ cup oat flour (or coconut flour)

1 cup carob powder

2 cups agave syrup

1 tablespoon vanilla extract

1 cup chopped walnuts

Directions

Preheat the oven to 325°F. Using Earth Balance buttery spread, generously grease a 13 x 9-inch pan.

Mix together the carob chips, Earth Balance, and tahini in a large heatproof bowl. Bring a medium saucepan filled halfway with water to a boil. Turn off the heat and place the bowl with the carob mixture over the hot water. Whisk the melting carob mixture until smooth.

Transfer the carob mixture to a stand-mixer bowl, and whisk in the avocado until incorporated. Whisk in the pureed beans until incorporated.

In a separate bowl or very large measuring cup, sift together the dry ingredients; mix thoroughly with a fork until all the dry ingredients are combined.

In a large measuring cup, combine the agave syrup with the vanilla.

On the mixer, switch to the paddle attachment. Alternate adding ½ cup at a time of the dry and agave mixtures to the batter. When the batter has been mixed well, fold in the walnuts. Let the batter rest until the oven has reached temperature.

When the oven has reached temperature, spread the batter into the prepared pan, making sure to get it into all the corners. It will be pretty thick. Bake for 40 minutes, or until a tester reveals a few moist crumbs. Let the brownies cool completely on a rack (at least 2 hours) before cutting into 48 pieces.

Nutrition Profile
110 calories, 4 g total fat, 0.5 g saturated fat, 0 mg cholesterol, 50 mg sodium, 20 g carbs, 2 g fiber, 2 g protein.

Spicy Biscotti

By Deb Schiff, author of the blog Altered Plates
alteredplates.blogspot.com

Deb's Rave—*Biscotti are reasonably easy to make, except for the fact that they are very time-consuming, due to the double baking. It's a good winter recipe because you can heat up your house as well as your tummy with these spicy, crunchy cookies.*

SERVINGS: 18 (2 COOKIES PER SERVING—1 COOKIE JUST ISN'T FAIR!)

Ingredients

2 tablespoons flaxseeds, ground

¼ cup water

1 cup whole wheat pastry flour

¼ cup barley flour (the original recipe called for coconut flour—go for it if you can find it!)

2 teaspoons baking powder

1 tablespoon ground cinnamon

2 tablespoons ground cardamom

1 tablespoon ground ginger

1 cup almond meal

⅔ cup agave syrup

1 teaspoon vanilla extract

1 tablespoon grated lemon zest

½ cup coarsely chopped almonds

Directions

Preheat the oven to 300°F. Line a baking sheet with parchment paper.

In a small bowl, combine the ground flaxseeds and the water, mixing well. Set aside.

In a large bowl, sift together the flours, baking powder, and spices. Mix in the almond meal until well incorporated.

In a medium bowl, beat together the agave syrup, vanilla, and lemon zest. Add the wet ingredients (including the flaxseed mixture) to the dry ingredients and stir until well combined. Fold in the almonds. Cover the dough with plastic wrap and refrigerate for 15 minutes.

Divide the dough in half. On a well-floured surface, shape each half into a log. Transfer the logs to the prepared baking sheet. There should be at least 3 inches between the logs. Lightly wet your hands with water and pat down the top of each log so that it is flattened a little.

Bake the logs for 30 minutes or until golden brown. Take the pan out of the oven and let the logs cool for 15 minutes on a wire rack. (Tip: Slide the entire thing, logs and parchment paper, onto the rack to cool.)

Transfer the logs one at a time to a cutting board and slice the logs into $\frac{1}{4}$-inch slices. Transfer the slices back to the baking sheet, relined with the same parchment paper, and bake them for 30 minutes, or until lightly browned. You want these to be crunchy, so don't be afraid if they darken a little. Just don't burn them. Transfer the cookies and the parchment paper to a wire rack and let the cookies cool completely before serving.

Nutrition Profile
130 calories, 5 g total fat, 0 g saturated fat, 0 mg cholesterol, 50 mg sodium, 19 g carbs, 3 g fiber, 3 g protein.

Pan-Cooked Apples and Pears in Grape Juice

Courtesy of Welch's
www.welchs.com

Welch's Tips—*This is great as a topping for cake, yogurt, or ice cream.*

SERVINGS: 6

Ingredients
2 cooking apples (Golden Delicious or Granny Smith), peeled, cored, and cut into chunks
2 Bosc pears, peeled, cored, and cut into chunks
2 tablespoons freshly squeezed lemon juice

1 tablespoon low-fat margarine

¼ cup sugar

1 orange

1 cinnamon stick, broken into pieces

⅔ cup Welch's purple grape juice

1 cup fresh or frozen blueberries

1 teaspoon cornstarch

2 tablespoons water

1 fresh mint sprig, for garnish

Directions

In a bowl, toss the apples and pears with the lemon juice, to prevent discoloring.

In a skillet over low heat, melt the margarine, add the sugar, and stir to form a paste. Stir in the fruit chunks, and cook for 2 minutes, or until well coated in the sugar paste.

Pare off a few strips of orange peel and add to the pan along with the cinnamon pieces. Add the grape juice, then extract the juice from the orange and pour it into the pan. Bring to a boil, reduce the heat, and simmer, stirring occasionally, for 10 minutes. Add the blueberries. Cook for 5 minutes, or until the apples and pears are tender.

Dissolve the cornstarch in the water and add to the mixture. Cook for 1 minute. Remove from the heat. Discard the orange peel and cinnamon pieces. Transfer the fruit to a serving plate. Garnish with a sprig of fresh mint and serve hot or cold.

Nutrition Profile

150 calories, 2 g total fat, 0 g saturated fat, 0 mg cholesterol, 25 mg sodium, 36 g carbs, 4 g fiber, 1 g protein.

Summer Fruits Pie

By Deb Schiff, author of the blog Altered Plates
alteredplates.blogspot.com

Deb's Tips—*Making this pie (like making any good pie) requires a serious time commitment. You can make the crust in advance and either freeze or refrigerate it for several days. The filling also may be made a day or two in advance. To make a fall seasonal pie, use more apples and pears with the cranberries, and omit the other berries.*

SERVINGS: 10

Ingredients

Crust
2 cups rolled oats
¾ cup walnuts
½ cup barley flour
½ cup whole wheat pastry flour
1 teaspoon apple pie spice
½ stick Earth Balance buttery spread, cut into ½-inch cubes and frozen for 1 hour
2 tablespoons agave syrup

Filling
⅔ cup cranberries
1 cup pitted cherries
1 cup blueberries
1 cup sliced strawberries
2 small pears, peeled, cored, and sliced thin

1 small apple, peeled, cored, and sliced thin

1 small nectarine, peeled, pitted, and sliced thin

Juice of $\frac{1}{2}$ lemon

$\frac{1}{4}$ cup agave syrup

$\frac{1}{4}$ cup cornstarch

Topping

$1\frac{1}{2}$ cups rolled oats

1 teaspoon ground cinnamon

2 tablespoons Earth Balance buttery spread

2 tablespoons agave syrup

Directions

Crust: Pour the oats and walnuts into a food processor and blend until the walnut pieces are $\frac{1}{8}$ inch or smaller. Add the barley flour, whole wheat pastry flour, and apple pie spice. Process for 30 seconds more. Add the frozen Earth Balance cubes and process until they are incorporated into the flours. While the processor is on, add the agave syrup and blend just until the syrup has been incorporated. Remove the dough from the processor, scooping it onto a large piece of plastic wrap. Fold the plastic up around the dough and gently shape the dough into a disk. Refrigerate the dough for at least 1 hour. Once the dough has been chilled, press it into a 9-inch pie dish, cover with plastic wrap, and refrigerate for at least 1 hour more.

Filling: Combine all the filling ingredients and mix well. Let sit for at least 1 hour. Once the filling has rested, pour it into the chilled piecrust and wrap and refrigerate the pie until the topping is prepared.

Topping: In a large bowl, combine the oats and cinnamon. Using your fingers, mix the Earth Balance buttery spread into the oats. It should look a bit clumpy. Drizzle the agave syrup over the mixture and combine well. Let the mixture sit until you're ready to top the pie.

To Bake: Preheat the oven to 350°F. Take the pie out of the refrigerator and press the topping onto the top of the pie, then move the pie to a rimmed baking sheet lined with parchment paper (this is just in case the pie bubbles over). Bake the pie at 350°F for 15 minutes; take it out, reduce the oven temperature to 325°F, and tent the pie with aluminum foil. Bake the pie for 40 minutes, then uncover and bake for 15 minutes more, or until golden brown.

Nutrition Profile
390 calories, 15 g total fat, 3.5 g saturated fat, 0 mg cholesterol, 75 mg sodium, 61 g carbs, 8 g fiber, 8 g protein.

ENTRÉES

Christine's Yummy Bean and Cheese Tostada

By Christine Gerbstadt, MD, RD
www.nutronicsinc.com

SERVINGS: 2

Ingredients
½ cup mashed cooked pinto beans (drain if using canned)
2 (6-inch) corn tostadas
½ cup grated Monterey Jack cheese
½ cup shredded romaine lettuce
¼ cup tomato salsa

Directions
Warm the beans and spread them equally on top of the tostadas.
Spread ¼ cup of cheese, ¼ cup of lettuce, and 2 tablespoons of
salsa on each. Eat and enjoy!

Nutrition Profile
260 calories, 10 g total fat, 5 g saturated fat, 30 mg cholesterol, 460 mg sodium, 49 g carbs, 6 g fiber, 26 g protein.

Irish Poached Salmon

By Chef J. Hugh McEvoy (aka "Chef J")
www.researchchefs.us

Chef J's Rave—*This is a nice change from everyday baked or grilled salmon!*

SERVINGS: 4

Ingredients
½ cup low-sodium chicken broth
½ cup dry white wine
½ cup skim milk
1 tablespoon diced shallot
1 lemon slice
1 fresh dill sprig
¼ teaspoon sea salt
4 (6-ounce) salmon fillets
Garnishes

Directions
Combine the broth, wine, and milk in a deep pan. Heat to barely simmering (170°F). Add the shallot, lemon slice, dill sprig, salt, and salmon. Cover and simmer for about 15 minutes, until the salmon is opaque and cooked fully. Discard the poaching ingredients before serving.

Serve hot with Greek-style yogurt, lemon, and chopped fresh dill. This dish may be chilled and served cold at brunch.

Nutrition Profile
350 calories, 18 g total fat, 3.5 g saturated fat, 100 mg cholesterol, 270 mg sodium, 3 g carbs, 0 g fiber, 35 g protein.

Mediterranean Grilled Mackerel or Bluefish

By Chef J. Hugh McEvoy (aka "Chef J")
www.researchchefs.us

Chef J's Tip—*Almost any variety of fish will work well in this recipe. If you can't find mackerel or bluefish, salmon or tuna would work quite well.*

SERVINGS: 12

Ingredients

Sauce
½ teaspoon finely grated lemon zest
1½ tablespoons freshly squeezed lemon juice
Salt and pepper
⅓ cup extra-virgin olive oil
¼ cup pitted Kalamata olives, cut into slivers
3 tablespoons finely chopped fresh oregano, plus 6 large sprigs

1 (3¼- to 3½-pound) cleaned whole bluefish, Spanish mackerel, or striped bass
2 tablespoons olive oil
Salt and pepper
6 (¼-inch-thick) lemon slices

Directions

Lightly oil the grill rack. Preheat the grill to 450°F, or to medium hot if using a charcoal grill or a grill that doesn't have a thermostat. Whisk together the zest, lemon juice, and salt and pepper to taste, then add the olive oil in a stream, whisking until well combined. Whisk in the olives and chopped oregano. Set the sauce aside.

Make 1-inch-long slits at 2-inch intervals down the middle of the fish on both sides with a sharp paring knife, and then brush the fish all over with the 2 tablespoons olive oil and season with salt and pepper.

Season the fish cavity with salt and pepper, then evenly distribute 3 lemon rounds and 3 oregano sprigs in the cavity. Close the cavity, and then evenly arrange the remaining 3 lemon rounds and 3 oregano sprigs on top of the fish. Tie the fish closed with kitchen string at 2-inch intervals, securing the lemon slices and oregano sprigs to the fish.

Grill the fish, covering it only if using a gas grill, for 15 minutes. Turn the fish over using a metal spatula and tongs, then grill until just cooked through, about 15 minutes more. Transfer the fish to a large platter using two metal spatulas, then cut and discard the string. Serve the fish with the sauce.

Nutrition Profile

250 calories, 15 g total fat, 2.5 saturated fat, 80 mg cholesterol, 130 mg sodium, 0 g carbs, 0 g fiber, 27 g protein.

Chicken Thighs with Red Wine, Dried Plums, and Garlic

By Chef Elizabeth Wiley, from the Meadowlark Restaurant
in Dayton, Ohio
www.meadowlarkrestaurant.com

Dave's Tip—*I was really concerned about the fat content of this dish, but was happy to see that the saturated fat wasn't that high after all. The analysis was with the skin and all, so avoiding the skin will reduce it even more! Chef Wiley refers to herself as the "thigh evangelist." I have officially become a believer!*

SERVINGS: 4

Ingredients
8 pitted dried plums (or more to taste)
8 cloves garlic, peeled (or more to taste)
2 whole cloves
½ cinnamon stick, bashed with a pestle
1 fresh rosemary sprig, bashed with a pestle
8 chicken thighs
½ cup low-sodium chicken broth
Juice of ½ orange
¾ cup dry red wine
Salt and pepper

Directions
Preheat the oven to 325°F.

Scatter the dried plums, garlic cloves, cloves, cinnamon pieces, and rosemary in the bottom of a roasting pan. Arrange the chicken thighs on top, skin side up. Mix the broth, orange juice, and red wine together. Pour over the chicken. Salt and pepper the chicken skin well. Cover the pan with aluminum foil. Bake for 2 hours. Let the chicken rest in the juices for 10 to 15 minutes.

Remove the chicken to a platter or individual plates. Gently pick out the dried plums and garlic cloves, and serve one of each per piece of chicken. Strain the juices and ladle off the fat. Check for seasoning, adjusting with salt and pepper if necessary. Serve the chicken, dried plums, roasted garlic, and juices with mashed or boiled potatoes and steamed kale, green beans, turnips, or any other vegetable you like!

Nutrition Facts
310 calories, 11 g total fat, 3g saturated fat, 100 mg cholesterol, 150 mg sodium, 16 g carbs, 2 g fiber, 29 g protein.

Grilled Chicken Salad with Pomegranate Vinaigrette and Mango Gelée Garnish

By Executive Chef Don Zajac, from Phil Stefani Signature Restaurants
www.stefanirestaurants.com

Servings: 1

Mango Gelée
3 gelatin leaves
2 cups cold water
2 cups mango juice

Pomegranate Vinaigrette
½ cup pomegranate juice
1 teaspoon honey

1 teaspoon minced shallot

1 tablespoon rice wine vinegar

3 teaspoons freshly squeezed lime juice

$\frac{1}{4}$ teaspoon minced jalapeño pepper

2 tablespoons extra-virgin olive oil

Kosher salt and white pepper

Salad

4 ounces skinless chicken tenderloins

1 teaspoon extra-virgin olive oil

$\frac{1}{4}$ teaspoon kosher salt

1 dash pepper

2 tablespoons pomegranate vinaigrette

1 cup mesclun greens

1 tablespoon sunflower seeds, shelled and toasted in a dry skillet, for garnish

$\frac{1}{4}$ cup mango gelée, diced, for garnish

Directions

Mango Gelée: Line a half sheet pan with plastic wrap. "Bloom" the gelatin leaves in the cold water until softened. In a small saucepan, heat the mango juice to 120°F. Remove the leaves from the water and squeeze to remove the excess liquid. Add the leaves to the mango juice and stir until dissolved. Pour the mixture onto the prepared sheet pan and place in the refrigerator until set (about 2 to 3 hours). Slice the gelée into small dice. Set aside in the refrigerator.

Pomegranate Vinaigrette: In a saucepan, combine the pomegranate juice, honey, and shallot. Bring to a simmer and reduce the mixture to 2 tablespoons; strain and let cool. In a mixing bowl, combine the reduction with the vinegar, lime juice, and jalapeño and whisk slowly, adding the olive oil to create an emulsion. Season to taste with the salt and white pepper.

Salad: Preheat the grill to 450°F (gas grill) or medium high (other grill). Season the chicken tenderloins with the olive oil, salt, and pepper; grill to an internal temperature of 165°F. Slice the chicken into bite-sized pieces. In a mixing bowl, combine the 2 tablespoons of the vinaigrette with the mesclun greens and chicken. Plate the salad, then garnish with the toasted sunflower seeds and the ¼ cup of the diced mango gelée.

Reserved mango gelée and pomegranate dressing will keep up to two weeks in sealed containers in the refrigerator. Add them as a topping over salads, fruits, and vegetable and grain sides. Be creative!

Nutrition Profile
300 calories, 13 g total fat, 2 g saturated fat, 65 mg cholesterol, 580 mg sodium, 15 g carbs, 2 g fiber, 29 g protein.

Moroccan Vegetable Stew with California Dried Plums

Courtesy of the California Dried Plum Board
www.californiadriedplums.org

Dave's Tip—*You can substitute whole wheat couscous or brown rice for the quinoa.*

SERVINGS: 6

Ingredients
2 cups quinoa
2 tablespoons extra-virgin olive oil

1 large onion, cut into ½-inch crescents

½ teaspoon ground cinnamon

½ teaspoon ground ginger

½ teaspoon sweet paprika

¼ teaspoon saffron threads

1 (1-pound) butternut squash, peeled, seeded, and cut into 1-inch cubes

2 small fennel bulbs, trimmed and cut into ½-inch-wide strips

1 (14.5-ounce) can diced tomatoes, with juice

½ teaspoon salt

1½ cups pitted California dried plums

¼ cup chopped fresh cilantro

Directions

Rinse the quinoa in a fine-mesh strainer. Place in a saucepan with 4 cups water. Bring to a simmer and reduce the heat. Cover and cook for 15 to 20 minutes, until the water is absorbed. Set aside.

While the quinoa is cooking, in a large, deep skillet, heat the oil over medium heat. Add the onion, cinnamon, ginger, paprika, and saffron; cook, stirring, for about 5 minutes, until the onion begins to soften. Add the squash, fennel, tomatoes and juice, 1½ cups water, and salt. Cover and simmer for about 15 minutes, until the squash feels tender when pierced with a small sharp knife; add the dried plums and cook for 5 minutes more. (The stew may be cooked to this point up to 1 day ahead; refrigerate until needed, then reheat in a saucepan over low heat.) Just before serving, stir in the cilantro. Serve over the quinoa.

Nutrition Profile

400 calories, 8 g total fat, 1 g saturated fat, 0 mg cholesterol, 410 mg sodium, 74 g carbs, 11 g fiber, 12 g protein.

Dilled Salmon Cakes

Courtesy of Quaker Oats
www.quakeroats.com

SERVINGS: 5

Ingredients

Sauce
½ cup plain nonfat yogurt
⅓ cup chopped tomato
⅓ cup chopped peeled cucumber
1 tablespoon finely chopped onion
1 tablespoon finely chopped fresh dill

Salmon Cakes
1 (14¾-ounce) can pink salmon, drained and skin and bones removed
¾ cup Quaker oats (quick or old-fashioned)
⅓ cup nonfat milk
2 egg whites, lightly beaten
2 tablespoons finely chopped onion
1 tablespoon finely chopped fresh dill, or 1 teaspoon dried dill
¼ teaspoon salt (optional)

Directions
Sauce: Combine all the ingredients for the sauce in a small bowl; mix well. Cover and refrigerate while making the salmon cakes.
Salmon Cakes: Combine all the ingredients for the salmon cakes in a medium bowl; mix well. Let stand for 5 minutes. Shape into 5 oval patties about 1 inch thick. Lightly spray a nonstick skillet

with nonstick cooking spray. Cook the salmon cakes over medium heat for 3 to 4 minutes on each side, until golden brown and heated through. Serve with the sauce.

Nutrition Profile
180 calories, 6 g total fat, 1 g saturated fat, 30 mg cholesterol, 400 mg sodium, 12 g carbs, 2 g fiber, 19 g protein.

Polenta Pizza

By Veronica "Roni" Noone
www.greenlitebites.com

Dave's Tip—*This is a great spin on traditional pizza that uses polenta as the crust. To make life easier, I like using pre-made polenta that comes in a tube shape. That way, when you slice it crosswise, you already have the crust shape!*

SERVINGS: 6

Ingredients
6 ($\frac{1}{4}$-inch-thick) polenta slices
6 tablespoons pizza sauce
1 teaspoon garlic powder
1 tablespoon chopped fresh basil
$\frac{1}{2}$ cup grated mozzarella cheese
$\frac{1}{4}$ cup grated Parmesan cheese
$\frac{1}{2}$ teaspoon pepper

Directions
Preheat the broiler.

Cook the polenta slices in a nonstick skillet sprayed with non-stick cooking spray over medium-high heat for 3 to 4 minutes a side, until just browning.

Top each cooked polenta "crust" with a smear of pizza sauce, and sprinkle with the garlic powder. Add the basil, then sprinkle with the cheeses and pepper.

Broil for about 2 minutes, until the cheeses melt.

Nutrition Profile
180 calories, 8 g total fat, 4.5 g saturated fat, 25 mg cholesterol, 690 mg sodium, 18 g carbs, 1 g fiber, 11 g protein.

Cocoa-Encrusted Salmon with Blueberries

By Chef Jennifer Carden, author of The Toddler Café
www.thetoddlercafe.blogspot.com

SERVINGS: 4

Ingredients
4 cups water
2 Earl Grey tea bags (paper tags removed)
½ cup wild rice
¼ red onion, diced
1¼ teaspoons salt
1 pound salmon fillets
2 teaspoons unsweetened cocoa powder
1 teaspoon dry mustard
¾ cup fresh blueberries
½ cup slivered almonds, toasted in a dry skillet
1½ teaspoons extra-virgin olive oil

Directions

In a medium saucepan, boil the 4 cups water with the 2 tea bags. When the tea is at a rolling boil, remove the tea bags, discard, and add the rice, red onion, and 1 teaspoon of the salt. Simmer, uncovered, for 40 minutes.

While the rice is cooking, place the salmon on a lightly greased baking sheet. Mix together the cocoa powder, the remaining ¼ teaspoon salt, and the dry mustard, and spread the rub all over the fish with the back of a spoon or a pastry brush. Sprinkle the blueberries on the same baking sheet. Set aside.

When the rice is cooked, it will be split and curled over, and will be tender. When it is done, drain the rice, stir in the almonds, cover, and set aside.

Preheat the broiler. Set a rack in the top third of the oven.

Broil the fish until it is cooked through and the berries are warm, 6 to 10 minutes.

Place a scoop of rice on each plate, top with the fish and warm blueberries, and drizzle with the extra-virgin olive oil. Serve.

Nutrition Profile

270 calories, 9 g total fat, 1.5 g saturated fat, 60 mg cholesterol, 780 mg sodium, 20 g carbs, 2 g fiber, 26 g protein.

SANDWICHES

Roasted Vegetable and Sweet Swiss Panini

By Sue McCloskey, owner of Ponte Fresco Restaurant in Chicago
www.pontefrescousa.com

Sue's Tips—*I suggest using the delicious sweet Swiss cheese from Fair Oaks Farms (www.fofarms.com). This sandwich works great in a panini machine.*

SERVINGS: 4

Ingredients
1 tablespoon extra-virgin olive oil
8 asparagus spears
½ red onion, julienned
½ red bell pepper, julienned
½ large portobello mushroom, sliced thin

Salt and pepper

8 (½-inch-thick) slices crusty Italian whole grain bread

1 cup grated Fair Oaks sweet Swiss cheese (can substitute low-fat Swiss or mozzarella)

8 fresh basil leaves

Balsamic vinegar (optional)

Directions

Heat a griddle or sauté pan over medium-high heat. Drizzle the oil over the asparagus, onion, bell pepper, and mushroom, then sprinkle with salt and pepper to taste. Cook the vegetables until they are tender and grill marks appear, about 4 minutes per side. Remove from the heat.

Spray one side of each slice of bread with nonstick cooking spray. Place 1 slice of bread, sprayed side down, on the griddle. Immediately assemble the ingredients on top of the bread as follows: 2 tablespoons of cheese, 2 basil leaves, and one-fourth of the roasted vegetable mixture. Top with 2 tablespoons of cheese and 1 slice of bread with the sprayed side facing up. Cook on each side until browned or grill marks appear and the cheese is well melted. Repeat with the remaining bread and filling to make 3 more sandwiches. Serve with small bowls of balsamic vinegar for dipping, if desired.

Nutrition Profile

250 calories, 7 g total fat, 2 g saturated fat, 10 mg cholesterol, 298 mg sodium, 29 g carbs, 6 g fiber, 17 g protein.

Healthy Turkey Salad Pocket

Courtesy of the California Dried Plum Board
www.californiadriedplums.org

SERVINGS: 6

Ingredients
2 cups diced cooked turkey or chicken
¾ cup quartered pitted dried plums
½ cup chopped celery
½ cup plain nonfat yogurt
¼ cup chopped scallions
1 tablespoon sweet hot mustard
Salt and pepper
6 lettuce leaves
3 whole wheat pita breads, halved

Directions
In a medium bowl, combine the turkey, dried plums, celery, yogurt, scallions, and mustard until thoroughly mixed. Season to taste with salt and pepper. Cover and store in the refrigerator for up to 3 days. To serve, insert 1 lettuce leaf and spoon ½ cup of the mixture into each pita pocket.

Nutrition Profile
233 calories, 2 g total fat, 1 g saturated fat, 33 mg cholesterol, 357 mg sodium, 35 g carbs, 4 g fiber, 19 g protein.

BREAKFAST

Capp-oat-ccino Delight

By Jennette Fulda, author of Half-Assed: A Weight-Loss Memoir
and blogger at www.PastaQueen.com, courtesy of Quaker Oats

Jennette's Tip—*Save time in the morning by combining your
cup of coffee with a heart-healthy breakfast. Quick and easy,
this recipe will give you a shot of energy that will also keep you
going until lunchtime.*

SERVINGS: 1

Ingredients
¾ cup Quaker quick oats
2 teaspoons instant coffee
1 tablespoon agave syrup

¼ cup skim milk
½ cup water

Directions
Combine the Quaker quick oats, instant coffee, and agave syrup. Mix in the skim milk and water. Microwave the mixture for 1 minute and 45 seconds. Enjoy!

Nutrition Profile
340 calories, 4.5 g total fat, 0 g saturated fat, 0 mg cholesterol, 40 mg sodium, 63 g carbs, 7 g fiber, 12 g protein.

Raspberry-Yogurt Muffins

Courtesy of the Washington Red Raspberry Commission
www.raspberryinfo.com

SERVINGS: 12

Dave's Tips—*Adding raspberry yogurt gives double the raspberry flavor and a wonderful texture to these easy muffins. No need to thaw the raspberries—just toss them in right from the freezer. And, if you wish, you can glaze the muffins with confectioners' sugar mixed with a little lemon juice.*

Ingredients
1¾ cups all-purpose flour
⅓ cup sugar
1 teaspoon baking powder
½ teaspoon baking soda

½ teaspoon salt

6 ounces raspberry nonfat yogurt

⅓ cup canola oil

1 egg

1 cup frozen Washington raspberries

Directions

Preheat the oven to 400°F. Spray, grease, or put paper liners in twelve 2¾-inch muffin cups.

In a medium mixing bowl, stir together the dry ingredients. In a small bowl, beat together the yogurt, oil, and egg. Stir the yogurt mixture into the dry mixture until almost blended. Add the raspberries and stir until the batter is just blended. Do not overmix. Spoon into the prepared muffin cups. Bake until nicely browned, about 20 minutes.

Nutrition Profile

160 calories, 7 g total fat, 1 g saturated fat, 18 mg cholesterol, 185 mg sodium, 22 g carbs, 1 g fiber, 3 g protein.

Zucchini-Cranberry Muffins

By Deb Schiff, author of the blog Altered Plates
alteredplates.blogspot.com

Deb's Tip—*This recipe uses avocado to replace most of the fat found in traditional muffin recipes. You get all the buttery flavor without the bad fats. If you're in a bind for time or you do not have a blender, you can use a whisk to mash and whip the avocado.*

SERVINGS: 12

Ingredients

1½ cups whole wheat pastry flour

¼ cup barley flour

1 teaspoon baking powder

1 teaspoon baking soda

½ teaspoon ground cinnamon

½ teaspoon ground nutmeg

¼ teaspoon salt

½ cup chopped walnuts

⅔ cup agave syrup

2 tablespoons extra-virgin olive oil

½ cup whipped avocado (easily done in a blender or with an immersion blender)

½ teaspoon vanilla extract

¼ teaspoon *fiori di Sicilia* extract (optional)

1⅓ cups grated zucchini (leave the skin on for lovely green bits)

½ cup frozen cranberries

Directions

Preheat the oven to 325°F. Line two muffin pans with nice paper liners.

Sift together the dry ingredients (except the walnuts) into a large bowl with a lip or into a very large measuring cup. Fold in the walnuts, making sure to mix them in well. They also help to better distribute all the dry ingredients.

In a separate large bowl, whisk together the agave syrup, olive oil, avocado, vanilla, and *fiori di Sicilia,* if desired, until well blended. Ensure that there are no lumps of avocado. With a big spoon or silicone spatula, mix in the zucchini. Add the dry ingredients, mixing until just blended. Fold in the cranberries for about 1 minute.

Using an ice cream scoop, fill the muffin liners. The muffins will rise a little, so make sure not to overfill the liners. Bake for 12 minutes, then rotate the pans and bake for another 12 minutes or until a bamboo tester comes out clean. The tops should be golden brown.

Let the muffins rest in their pans for 10 minutes, no more. Then remove them from the pans to cool completely on wire racks. Break 'em open and enjoy!

Nutrition Profile
190 calories, 7 g total fat, 1 g saturated fat, 0 mg cholesterol, 190 mg sodium, 31 g carbs, 4 g fiber, 3 g protein.

Crumb-Topped Georgia Pecan and Cherry Cereal Bars

Courtesy of the Georgia Pecan Commission
www.georgiapecansfit.org

Georgia Pecan Commission's Tip—*Other fruit spreads, such as raspberry and blueberry, can easily be substituted.*

SERVINGS: 12

Ingredients
1 cup whole wheat flour
1 cup quick-cooking oats
1 cup puffed rice cereal (preferably brown rice)
1 cup chopped Georgia pecans
1 teaspoon ground cinnamon
½ teaspoon baking powder

½ teaspoon salt

4 tablespoons (½ stick) unsalted butter, softened

2 tablespoons canola oil

⅓ cup packed light brown sugar

1 teaspoon vanilla extract

1 (10-ounce) jar tart cherry fruit spread

Directions

Preheat the oven to 350°F. Butter a 9-inch square baking pan.

In a medium bowl, combine the flour, oats, puffed rice, pecans, cinnamon, baking powder, and salt. Set aside.

In a large bowl, beat the butter, oil, brown sugar, and vanilla until blended and creamy. Add the dry ingredients and mix until moistened and a crumbly dough forms. Reserve 1½ cups of the dough for the topping. Press the remaining dough evenly into the bottom of the prepared pan.

Spread the cherry fruit spread evenly over the dough in the pan. Sprinkle the reserved dough mixture over the top, leaving some random spaces where the fruit is uncovered. Gently press down to adhere the topping to the fruit layer. Bake for 30 minutes, or until the topping is a deep golden color. When cooled to warm, slice into twelve 3 x 2-inch bars.

Nutrition Profile

216 calories, 11 g total fat, 3 g saturated fat, 10 mg cholesterol, 132 mg sodium, 22 g carbs, 3 g fiber, 3 g protein.

Powerhouse Dried Plum Bars

Courtesy of the California Dried Plum Board
www.californiadriedplums.org

SERVINGS: 16

Ingredients
1½ cups coarsely chopped pitted dried plums
⅓ cup apricot jam
2 cups rolled oats (quick or old-fashioned)
¾ cup packed light brown sugar
½ cup all-purpose flour
½ teaspoon ground cinnamon
½ teaspoon salt
½ teaspoon baking soda
1 egg
1½ tablespoons unsalted butter or margarine, melted
Confectioners' sugar (optional)

Directions
Preheat the oven to 350°F. Lightly spray an 8-inch square baking pan with nonstick cooking spray.

In a medium bowl, combine the dried plums and apricot jam; set aside. In a large bowl, combine the oats, brown sugar, flour, cinnamon, salt, and baking soda; mix well. Lightly beat together the egg and butter; add to the oat mixture, mixing until crumbly. Press 2 cups of the mixture into the bottom of the prepared pan. Spread the dried plum mixture over the oats; sprinkle the remaining oat mixture over the top. Bake for 20 to 22 minutes, until deep golden brown. Let cool in the pan on a wire rack. Sprinkle with confectioners' sugar, if desired; cut into 16 bars.

Nutrition Profile
200 calories, 3 g fat, 0 g saturated fat, 15 mg cholesterol, 135 mg sodium, 39 g carbs, 3 g fiber, 4 g protein.

Georgia Pecan Muesli

By Chef Scott Peacock, courtesy of the Georgia Pecan Commission
www.georgiapecansfit.org

SERVINGS: 6

Ingredients
2 cups old-fashioned rolled oats
1 cup chopped pecans
$\frac{1}{2}$ cup oat bran
$\frac{1}{4}$ cup packed light brown sugar
$\frac{1}{4}$ cup golden raisins
$\frac{1}{4}$ cup diced dried figs
$\frac{1}{4}$ cup diced dates
$\frac{1}{4}$ teaspoon salt
Yogurt or milk, to serve
Fresh fruit (optional)
Honey (optional)

Directions
Combine all the measured ingredients and mix well. Serve with yogurt or milk and fresh fruit, such as a banana, if desired.

For a softer, creamier texture, yogurt or milk may be stirred into the muesli and refrigerated overnight before serving. If desired, drizzle with a little honey before eating.

Nutrition Profile (without yogurt, milk, fresh fruit, or honey)
360 calories, 13 g total fat, 1 g saturated fat, 0 mg cholesterol, 93
mg sodium, 54 g carbs, 7 g fiber, 8 g protein.

Soufflé Omelet with Balsamic Strawberries

Courtesy of the California Strawberry Commission
www.calstrawberry.com

SERVINGS: 2

Ingredients
8 ounces fresh California strawberries, hulled and quartered
1 tablespoon chopped fresh mint
1 tablespoon aged balsamic vinegar
2 teaspoons granulated sugar
2 large eggs, separated
¼ teaspoon vanilla extract
2 teaspoons unsalted butter
Confectioners' sugar

Directions
In a medium bowl, combine the strawberries, mint, balsamic
vinegar, and 1½ teaspoons of the granulated sugar; set aside.

In a small bowl, whisk the egg yolks with the vanilla and the
remaining ½ teaspoon granulated sugar for 1 minute, or until
slightly thickened.

In the bowl of an electric mixer, beat the egg whites until they
form soft peaks. With a rubber spatula, fold the yolks into the
whites until no streaks remain.

In a 10-inch nonstick skillet over medium heat, melt the butter. (To make 2 individual omelets, use a 6-inch nonstick skillet.) When the butter is sizzling, add the egg mixture, spreading it into an even layer with the spatula. Cover the pan; reduce the heat to low. Cook the omelet for 3 to 4 minutes, until golden brown on the bottom and barely set on top. Spoon the strawberry mixture down the center of the omelet; with a clean rubber spatula, fold the omelet in half over the filling. Slide the omelet onto a plate; dust with confectioners' sugar.

Nutrition Profile
160 calories, 9 g total fat, 4 g saturated fat, 225 mg cholesterol, 70 mg sodium, 15 g carbs, 3 g fiber, 7 g protein.

Triple-Grain Georgia Pecan Pancakes

Courtesy of the Georgia Pecan Commission
www.georgiapecansfit.org

Georgia Pecan Commission's Tip—*You can feel free to make flour substitutions here, switching buckwheat flour or oat flour for the soy or cornmeal in the recipe.*

SERVINGS: 4 (2 PANCAKES PER SERVING)

Ingredients

Dry Mix (Makes About 4½ Cups)
1 cup whole wheat pastry flour
1 cup all-purpose flour
½ cup yellow cornmeal

½ cup soy flour

½ cup maple sugar, or ¼ cup granulated sugar

2½ teaspoons baking powder

1 teaspoon baking soda

1 teaspoon salt

1½ cups chopped pecans

Wet Ingredients (for ¾ Cup of Dry Mix)

½ cup low-fat milk

1 large egg

1 tablespoon freshly squeezed lemon juice

1 tablespoon vegetable oil

Maple syrup, to serve

Directions

Combine all the dry ingredients in a resealable 6-cup container; mix very well to blend evenly. If not using within a week, refrigerate the dry mixture.

To make eight 3-inch pancakes, heat an oiled skillet or griddle over medium-high heat. Beat together the milk, egg, lemon juice, and vegetable oil until blended. Stir in ¾ cup dry mix, mixing just until a smooth batter forms. When the skillet is hot (a sprinkle of water will dance and steam on the surface), pour a scant ¼ cup batter into the pan for each pancake and cook for 2 to 3 minutes per side. Serve the pancakes warm with maple syrup.

Nutrition Profile (per two 3-inch pancakes, without maple syrup)

188 calories, 4.5 g total fat, 1 g saturated fat, 54 mg cholesterol, 72 mg sodium, 18 g carbs, 2 g fiber, 6 g protein.

Cherry-Chai Spice Granola

By Deb Schiff, author of the blog Altered Plates
alteredplates.blogspot.com

SERVINGS: 30

Ingredients
3 cups rolled oats
¾ cup barley flour
¾ cup shredded unsweetened dried coconut (as finely shredded as possible)
¾ cup chopped almonds
¾ cup chopped pecans
¼ cup sesame seeds
½ cup flaxseeds, ground
¾ cup sunflower seeds
½ cup pumpkin seeds or pepitas
1 teaspoon ground cinnamon
1 teaspoon ground ginger
1 teaspoon ground allspice
1 teaspoon ground nutmeg
1 teaspoon ground cardamom
⅓ cup grapeseed oil
1 cup agave syrup
1 tablespoon vanilla extract

Postbaking Add-Ins
¾ cup apple juice–sweetened dried cranberries
¾ cup unsweetened dried cherries
¾ cup chopped pitted dried plums

Directions

Preheat the oven to 325°F. Line two rimmed baking sheets with parchment paper.

In your largest bowl, combine the first fourteen ingredients (all the ingredients up until the oil). Ensure that there aren't any flour pockets.

In a much smaller bowl, blend the three wet ingredients until well incorporated.

Add the wet ingredients to the dry ingredients and mix until all the dry ingredients have been coated. Spread the mixture equally onto the prepared baking sheets. Wash and dry the bowl and set aside.

Bake for 15 minutes, then take the sheets out of the oven, stir the granola, and switch the positions of the sheets (the top one goes on the middle rack and vice versa). Bake the granola for another 15 minutes. Stir once more, and then bake until uniformly lightly browned. It won't take more than another 15 minutes—keep an eye on it, or you may burn it. If you like a chunkier granola, stir it less.

During the final baking, combine the add-ins in your largest bowl. When the granola is done baking, immediately slide it off the pans on top of the add-ins in the bowl and stir well. Spread the mixture into the pans and let the pans cool on top of wire racks for at least 2 hours before transferring the granola to airtight containers.

Nutrition Profile

240 calories, 13 g total fat, 2.5 g saturated fat, 0 mg cholesterol, 20 mg sodium, 27 g carbs, 4 g fiber, 5 g protein.

Creamy Cherry Oatmeal

By Sharon Grotto

SERVINGS: 4

Ingredients
2 cups 2% milk
1 cup water
1 cup rolled oats
½ cup dried tart cherries
2 teaspoons vanilla extract
¼ teaspoon ground cinnamon
⅛ teaspoon grated nutmeg
⅛ teaspoon salt
Honey, light brown sugar, or maple syrup to taste

Directions
Place all the ingredients in a medium saucepan. Simmer over medium heat, stirring occasionally, for 10 to 13 minutes, until the desired creaminess is achieved.

Nutrition Profile
210 calories, 4 g total fat, 1.5 g saturated fat, 10 mg cholesterol, 150 mg sodium, 35 g carbs, 2 g fiber, 8 g protein.

Chef Wiley's Granola

By Chef Elizabeth Wiley, from the Meadowlark Restaurant
in Dayton, Ohio
www.meadowlarkrestaurant.com

SERVINGS: 8 TO 10

Ingredients
4 cups rolled oats
¾ cup sliced or coarsely chopped assorted raw nuts
½ cup packed light brown sugar
¼ teaspoon salt
⅛ teaspoon ground cinnamon
⅓ cup canola oil
¼ cup honey
2 tablespoons granulated sugar
4 teaspoons vanilla extract

Directions
Position a rack in the middle of the oven and preheat the oven to 325°F. Lightly spray a baking sheet with nonstick cooking spray.

Mix the oats, nuts, brown sugar, salt, and cinnamon in a large bowl. Combine the oil, honey, and granulated sugar in a small saucepan. Bring to a simmer over medium heat. Remove from the heat and stir in the vanilla. Pour the hot liquid over the oat mixture and stir very well to coat completely. Don't miss any spots!

Spread the granola out on the prepared baking sheet. Bake, stirring every 5 to 7 minutes, for about 30 minutes, until deep golden brown. Let the granola cool completely before breaking it up and storing in an airtight container.

Nutrition Profile
290 calories, 15 g total fat, 1 g saturated fat, 0 mg cholesterol, 60 mg sodium, 33 g carbs, 5 g fiber, 8 g protein.

Nutty Good Millet Muffins

By Chef Jennifer Carden, author of The Toddler Café
thetoddlercafe.blogspot.com

Jennifer's Tips—*When making muffins, start with room-temperature ingredients for a better end product. The less you mix and handle the batter, the more tender the muffin. If you can't find nut meals, just grind raw nuts in a food processor until they are the consistency of damp sand. The same goes for flaxseed meal—just grind flaxseeds in a blender if you can't find meal in the stores.*

SERVINGS: 12

Ingredients

Dry Ingredients
1½ cups whole wheat flour
½ cup hazelnut meal or almond meal
½ cup millet
½ teaspoon salt
1 tablespoon baking powder
½ teaspoon grated nutmeg

Wet Ingredients
2 eggs

1 cup buttermilk

⅔ cup light brown sugar

6 tablespoons (¾ stick) Earth Balance buttery spread, melted (set 1 tablespoon melted spread aside)

Topping

¼ cup light brown sugar

¼ cup hazelnut meal or almond meal

1 tablespoon flaxseed meal

Reserved 1 tablespoon melted Earth Balance buttery spread

Directions

Preheat the oven to 350°F. Move a rack to the middle of the oven. Line two muffin pans with paper liners or spray with nonstick cooking spray.

In a small bowl, whisk the dry ingredients together and set aside.

In a large bowl, combine the eggs, buttermilk, brown sugar, and 5 tablespoons of the melted Earth Balance spread. Whisk to combine. Add the dry ingredients and fold gently to combine. Drop by ice cream scoops into the muffin pans.

Mix the topping ingredients in a bowl and top each muffin with a teaspoon of topping, spreading it around to cover the top of the muffin. Bake for 15 minutes or until a toothpick comes out clean. Eat and enjoy!

Nutrition Profile

240 calories, 10 g total fat, 3 g saturated fat, 35 mg cholesterol, 300 mg sodium, 32 g carbs, 3 g fiber, 5 g protein.

SIDE DISHES

Japanese-Style Vegetable Fried Rice

By Chef Elizabeth Wiley, from the Meadowlark Restaurant
in Dayton, Ohio
www.meadowlarkrestaurant.com

SERVINGS: 6

Ingredients
2 tablespoons peanut or vegetable oil
1 tablespoon minced peeled fresh ginger
1 tablespoon minced garlic
1 cup sliced mushrooms
½ cup grated carrot
½ cup thinly sliced scallions
3 cups cooked rice
⅓ cup sake

1½ teaspoons low-sodium soy sauce
Salt and pepper
1 cup edamame (can also use cooked broccoli florets and/or cut-up green beans)
3 cups fresh spinach leaves

Directions
Put the oil, ginger, garlic, mushrooms, carrot, and scallions into a nonstick skillet and cook over medium heat until sizzling, stirring with a wooden spoon.

Add the cooked rice, stir, and cook for a few minutes. Make a hole in the rice to expose the bottom of the pan and pour the sake in, letting the sake start to come to a boil. Sprinkle in the soy sauce and salt and pepper. Toss to combine.

Add the edamame and the spinach leaves. Let the spinach wilt for a minute and toss to combine. Taste for salt and pepper.

Nutrition Profile
230 calories, 7 g total fat, 1 g saturated fat, 0 mg cholesterol, 100 mg sodium, 32 g carbs, 5 g fiber, 7 g protein.

Wild Mushroom Ris-oat-to

By Chef Spike Mendelsohn, courtesy of Quaker Oats
www.quakeroats.com

Chef Spike's Tips—*You can be creative and use any type of mushrooms you like, but I prefer using oysters or maitakes, as I feel they are more flavorful. Portobellos and buttons would also work just fine.*

SERVINGS: 6

Ingredients

Ris-oat-to
1½ cups water
2 (14-ounce) cans low-sodium chicken broth
Extra-virgin olive oil
1 cup diced yellow onions
1 clove garlic, minced
2 cups old-fashioned Quaker oats
1 cup dry white wine
1 cup freshly grated Parmigiano-Reggiano cheese
Sea salt and cracked black peppercorns

Mushrooms
2 tablespoons extra-virgin olive oil
4 cups sliced mushrooms of your choice
1 clove garlic, minced
½ teaspoon sea salt
½ teaspoon cracked black peppercorns
1 tablespoon chopped fresh thyme

Directions

Ris-oat-to: In a saucepan, bring the 1½ cups water and the broth to a simmer. Keep warm over medium heat. Heat a medium sauté pan over medium-high heat. Coat the pan with a drizzle of olive oil. Add the onions and garlic, and sauté for about 2 minutes, until golden brown. Add the oats, and toast until golden brown, stirring constantly. Add the wine; cook, stirring constantly, for 1 minute, or until the liquid is nearly absorbed. Stir in 1 cup of the broth mixture; cook, stirring constantly, for 4 minutes, or until the liquid is nearly absorbed. Add the remaining broth mixture, ½ cup at a time, stirring constantly until each portion of the broth mixture is absorbed before adding the next. Remove the ris-oat-to from the heat and add ½ cup of the cheese. Season with sea salt and cracked black pepper to taste.

Mushrooms: Heat the olive oil in a large nonstick skillet over medium-high heat. Add the mushrooms and garlic, and sauté for about 4 minutes, until the mushrooms are golden brown and crispy. At the last second, season with the salt, cracked black pepper, and fresh thyme.

To serve: Spoon the ris-oat-to into six bowls and top with the crispy mushrooms and the remaining ½ cup cheese.

Nutrition Profile

290 calories, 12 g total fat, 4 g saturated fat, 15 mg cholesterol, 320 mg sodium, 26 g carbs, 4 g fiber, 13 g protein.

Sharon's Moroccan Couscous

By Sharon Grotto

Sharon's Tip—*This can be served either hot as a side dish or cold as a refreshing, light salad.*

SERVINGS: 11

Ingredients
1½ cups water
8 ounces Israeli couscous
½ cup toasted and coarsely chopped walnuts
2 tablespoons lemon-infused extra-virgin olive oil
½ cup chopped carrot
16 ounces canned chickpeas, drained and rinsed
2 cloves garlic, minced
½ cup dried tart cherries (can substitute dried cranberries)
¼ cup chopped fresh parsley
2 teaspoons curry powder
½ teaspoon ground turmeric
½ teaspoon ground cinnamon
Salt and pepper

Directions
Preheat the oven to 350°F.

Bring the water to a boil in a medium saucepan; add the couscous. Cover the pan, reduce the heat, and simmer, stirring occasionally, for 8 to 10 minutes, until the water is absorbed. While the couscous is cooking, place the walnuts on a cookie sheet and bake for 8 to 10 minutes, checking frequently, until toasted, or light brown in color. Chop the walnuts and set them aside.

In a large sauté pan, heat the olive oil. Add the carrot, chickpeas, and garlic, and cook over medium heat for 3 to 4 minutes,
until the chickpeas have become slightly browned. Remove from
the heat. Add the cooked couscous, the toasted walnuts, and the
remaining ingredients and mix well. To serve cold, refrigerate
for at least 4 hours.

Nutrition Profile
210 calories, 6 g total fat, 1 g saturated fat, 0 mg cholesterol, 15
mg sodium, 32 g carbs, 4 g fiber, 6 g protein.

Roasted Autumn Vegetables in Sherry Sauce

By Chef Cheryl Bell, MS, RD, LDN, CHE

SERVINGS: 16

Ingredients
2 turnips
4 carrots
4 parsnips
4 Yukon gold potatoes
2 onions
1 small rutabaga
1 fennel bulb
3 tablespoons extra-virgin olive oil
¼ cup dry sherry
1 teaspoon dried thyme
Salt and pepper

Directions

Preheat the oven to 425°F.

Peel and/or trim all the vegetables and cut into bite-sized pieces. In a large bowl, toss the vegetables with the oil, sherry, thyme, and seasonings. Pour into a large casserole dish and cover with aluminum foil. Bake for about 1 hour, until the vegetables are tender when pierced with a fork.

Nutrition Profile

114 calories, 3 g total fat, 0 g saturated fat, 0 mg cholesterol, 32 mg sodium, 20 g carbs, 4 g fiber, 2 g protein.

Asparagus-Carrot Rolls

By Chef Justin Kubica, from CHOW restaurant in Elmhurst, Illinois
www.chowtogo.com

SERVINGS: 5 TO 6

Ingredients

1 large carrot

1 bunch asparagus

1½ teaspoons salt

2 tablespoons Dijon mustard

2 tablespoons honey

½ cup extra-virgin olive oil

Directions

Peel the carrot and cut off the ends. Trim the ends of the asparagus. Bring a large pot of water to a boil; add 1 teaspoon of the salt. Blanch the asparagus for 3 to 4 minutes, then remove with tongs and soak in ice water. Set aside. Using the same boiling water, cook the carrot until fork-tender, about 8 minutes, and add to the ice water. Once cooled, slice the carrot lengthwise into thin ribbons (about $\frac{1}{8}$ inch thick), using either a mandoline or a sharp knife. Lay each carrot ribbon out and roll 3 to 5 asparagus spears in the ribbon, wrapping the carrot around the middle of the spears. Lay attractively on a platter or individual plates.

In a bowl, combine the remaining $\frac{1}{2}$ teaspoon salt, the Dijon mustard, and the honey. Slowly whisk in the olive oil, and drizzle the dressing over the carrot rolls.

Nutrition Profile
210 calories, 19 g total fat, 2.5 g saturated fat, 0 mg cholesterol, 320 mg sodium, 9 g carbs, 1 g fiber, 1 g protein.

Asparagus-Sesame Stir-Fry

By Chef Carrie Walters, from Dorothy Lane Market in Dayton, Ohio
www.dorothylane.com

SERVINGS: 6

Ingredients
$1\frac{3}{4}$ pounds asparagus
2 teaspoons sugar
2 tablespoons low-sodium soy sauce
2 tablespoons chopped garlic
2 tablespoons sesame oil

4 teaspoons sesame seeds
1 teaspoon sea salt
1 teaspoon ground white pepper

Directions
Trim the ends off the asparagus. Cut on the bias into 2-inch pieces.

In a small bowl, mix the sugar with the soy sauce until the sugar is dissolved. Set aside.

Over high heat, sauté the garlic in a large skillet for 15 seconds in the sesame oil. Add the cut asparagus and stir-fry until crisp and tender, about 4 minutes. Add the soy sauce and sugar mixture, and toss all with the sesame seeds. Season with the salt and pepper.

Nutrition Profile
100 calories, 6 g total fat, 0.5 g saturated fat, 0 mg cholesterol, 460 mg sodium, 8 g carbs, 3 g fiber, 4 g protein.

Fingerling Potatoes with Asparagus

By Chef Carrie Walters, from Dorothy Lane Market in Dayton, Ohio
www.dorothylane.com

SERVINGS: 4

Ingredients
1 pound fingerling potatoes or other small potatoes, with skin on
½ teaspoon kosher salt

1 head garlic, roasted*
2 tablespoons chopped fresh tarragon
2 scallions, minced
1½ teaspoons balsamic vinegar
Pinch of red pepper flakes
Salt and pepper
¼ cup extra-virgin olive oil
1 pound asparagus, trimmed and blanched

Directions

Cover the potatoes with cold water in a small saucepan and add the kosher salt. Bring to a boil and then reduce the heat to a simmer and cook until the potatoes are tender, about 10 minutes. Drain and cover with cold water to stop the cooking process. Drain and place in a medium bowl.

In a small bowl, combine 2 teaspoons of the roasted garlic (or more to taste), the tarragon, scallions, balsamic vinegar, red pepper flakes, and salt and pepper to taste. Whisk in the olive oil and pour over the potatoes. Let stand for at least 15 minutes. Toss with the blanched asparagus. Serve warm or at room temperature.

Nutrition Profile

250 calories, 14 g total fat, 2 g saturated fat, 0 mg cholesterol, 250 mg sodium, 29 g carbs, 5 g fiber, 6 g protein.

To roast the garlic head, preheat the oven to 425°F. Halve the head horizontally. Place the halves, cut side up, on aluminum foil and drizzle with 1 to 2 teaspoons of olive oil and a splash of balsamic vinegar. Wrap in the foil and roast until soft, about 45 minutes. Let cool. Squeeze the pulp from the skins. Set aside until ready to use.

Roasted Root Vegetables

By Chef Carrie Walters, from Dorothy Lane Market in Dayton, Ohio
www.dorothylane.com

SERVINGS: 6

Ingredients
¼ cup extra-virgin olive oil
2 tablespoons pure maple syrup
1 clove garlic, minced
4 large beets, peeled and quartered
2 Yukon gold potatoes, quartered
2 carrots, peeled and cut diagonally into 2-inch-long pieces
2 parsnips, peeled and cut diagonally into 2-inch-long pieces
1 large sweet potato, peeled and cut into 1½-inch pieces
1 rutabaga, peeled and cut into 1½-inch pieces
1 large onion, peeled and quartered through the root end
Salt and pepper
2 tablespoons unsalted butter, melted
⅓ cup chopped scallions

Directions
Preheat the oven to 350°F.

Mix together the oil, syrup, and garlic in a small bowl. Place all the remaining ingredients except the seasonings, butter, and scallions on a large, heavy rimmed baking sheet. Pour the oil mixture over; toss to coat. Spread out the vegetables in a single layer. Sprinkle generously with salt and pepper. Bake, stirring occasionally, until tender and golden brown, about 1¼ hours. Transfer the vegetables to a platter. Drizzle the vegetables with the melted butter. Sprinkle with the chopped scallions, and serve immediately.

Nutrition Profile
240 calories, 10 g total fat, 3 g saturated fat, 10 mg cholesterol, 180 mg sodium, 36 g carbs, 8 g fiber, 4 g protein.

Vegetable Pavé with Cauliflower Coulis

By Executive Chef Don Zajac, from Phil Stefani Signature Restaurants
www.stefanirestaurants.com

SERVINGS: 16

Ingredients

Vegetable Pavé
1 pound Swiss chard, stems removed
½ cup low-sodium vegetable broth
1 tablespoon roasted-garlic olive oil
1 large Yukon gold potato, peeled and sliced thin
1 large sweet potato, peeled and sliced thin
1 large turnip, peeled and sliced thin
Kosher salt and white pepper

Cauliflower Coulis
8 ounces cauliflower florets
½ cup nonfat milk
1 clove garlic, crushed
¼ teaspoon kosher salt
¼ teaspoon white pepper

Turmeric Oil
¼ cup extra-virgin olive oil
½ teaspoon ground turmeric

Directions
Vegetable Pavé: Preheat the oven to 350°F. Steam the chard in the vegetable broth for 5 minutes; remove from the heat, let cool, and drain well. Coat the bottom and sides of an 8-inch square casserole dish with the roasted-garlic olive oil. Single-layer the Yukon gold, sweet potato, and turnip slices and the chard, seasoning each layer with salt and pepper. Repeat until the vegetables are used up. Cover with aluminum foil and, in order to compress the pavé so that it will slice without falling apart, place a slightly smaller baking dish on top. Bake for 2¼ hours; remove from the oven, take off the small baking dish and foil (taking care to avoid the hot steam), and let rest for 10 minutes.
Cauliflower Coulis: Simmer the florets with the milk and garlic for 10 minutes, or until tender. Drain, saving the poaching liquid. Puree the cauliflower and season with salt and pepper. If the puree is too thick, add a small amount of poaching liquid.
Tumeric Oil: Blend the olive oil and turmeric in a small saucepan. Simmer over medium heat just until aromatic. Remove from the heat and allow to infuse for 10 minutes.
To serve: Portion the pavé into 2-inch squares. Place 1 tablespoon of cauliflower coulis in the center of each plate. Place the pavé just off-center of the coulis. Drizzle with the turmeric oil.

Nutrition Profile
60 calories, 4.5 g total fat, 0.5 g saturated fat, 0 mg cholesterol, 125 mg sodium, 5 g carbs, 1 g fiber, 1 g protein.

Slow-Cooker Sweet Potatoes

By Veronica "Roni" Noone
www.greenlitebites.com

SERVINGS: 8

Ingredients

4 large sweet potatoes
1 tablespoon honey
1 tablespoon dark molasses
1 tablespoon balsamic vinegar
$\frac{1}{4}$ teaspoon ground allspice
Chopped fresh (or dried) parsley, for garnish

Directions

Scrub the potatoes. Cut into large chunks, leaving the skins on. Add the potatoes to a slow cooker.

In a small bowl, whisk together the honey, molasses, balsamic vinegar, and allspice, to make the marinade. Pour the marinade over the potatoes; stir to coat. Cover and cook on high for about 4 hours, until the potatoes are nice and soft. Serve in a casserole dish with a sprinkle of parsley.

Nutrition Profile

70 calories, 0 g total fat, 0 g saturated fat, 0 mg cholesterol, 35 mg sodium, 16 g carbs, 2 g fiber, 1 g protein.

Quinoa Pilaf with Currants and Turmeric

By Chef Elisa Hunziker
www.cancersurvivorchef.com

Chef Hunziker's Tip—*Can be served with chunks of cooked chicken or straight-up vegetarian by substituting veggie broth for the chicken broth.*

SERVINGS: 1

Ingredients
1 cup low-sodium chicken broth
1 cup freshly squeezed orange juice
1 cup quinoa, rinsed
½ teaspoon ground cumin
½ teaspoon ground turmeric
Grated zest of 1 orange
¼ cup dried currants
¼ cup pine nuts, toasted in a dry skillet
¼ cup chopped fresh cilantro
Salt and pepper
Mango chutney

Directions
Bring the chicken broth and orange juice to a boil and add the quinoa, cumin, and turmeric. Cover and cook over medium heat for 12 minutes, or until the quinoa has absorbed all the liquid.

While the quinoa is cooking, soak the currants in warm water. When the quinoa is done, fluff with a fork and stir in the orange zest, currants (drained), pine nuts, and cilantro. Season with salt and pepper to taste. Serve with mango chutney.

Nutrition Profile
320 calories, 4.5 g total fat, 0 g saturated fat, 10 mg cholesterol, 25 mg sodium, 67 g carbs, 10 g fiber, 8 g protein.

Curried Chickpeas and Kale

By Chef Cheryl Bell, MS, RD, LDN, CHE

Chef Bell's Tip—*You can substitute Swiss chard or frozen chopped spinach for the kale.*

SERVINGS: 6

Ingredients
2 tablespoons canola oil
1½ cups chopped onions
4 cloves garlic, minced
4 cups packed chopped kale
1½ teaspoons curry powder
1 teaspoon ground ginger
Salt
1½ cups low-sodium vegetable broth
3 cups cooked chickpeas, drained and rinsed if canned
1 cup chopped ripe tomato

Directions
In a 2-quart saucepan, heat the oil over medium heat. Add the onions and garlic and cook until softened, about 5 minutes. Add the kale. Cook, stirring occasionally, until softened, about 3 minutes. Stir in the curry powder, ginger, and salt to taste. Stir in the broth and bring to a boil. Add the chickpeas and tomato,

return to a boil, and then simmer, uncovered, for 25 minutes. Delicious served over brown rice.

Nutrition Profile
150 calories, 4 g total fat, 0 g saturated fat, 0 mg cholesterol, 245 mg sodium, 18 g carbs, 6 g fiber, 10 g protein.

SELECTED RESOURCES AND BIBLIOGRAPHY

For a complete listing of resources and references, go to www.101FoodsThatCouldSaveYourLife.com.

Part 1: The Skin You're In

Resources

National Institute of Arthritis and Musculoskeletal and Skin Diseases—www.niams.nih.gov

National Cancer Institute—www.nci.nih.gov

National Institutes of Health—www.nlm.nih.gov/medlineplus /eczema.html; www.nlm.nih.gov/medlineplus/psoriasis.html; www .nlm.nih.gov/medlineplus/print/acne.html

The American Academy of Dermatology—www.aad.org

www.skincarephysicians.com

www.emedicinehealth.com/eczema/article_em.htm

National Psoriasis Foundation—www.psoriasis.org/home

Mayo Clinic—www.mayoclinic.com/print/acne-treatments/SN00038 /METHOD=print; www.mayoclinic.com/health/dandruff

Nemours Foundation—http://kidshealth.org/teen/your_body/beautiful /prevent_acne.html

Medicine Net—www.medicinenet.com/seborrhea/article.htm

Bibliography

Adebamowo CA, et al. High school dietary dairy intake and teenage acne. *J Am Acad Dermatol.* 2005 Feb;52(2):207–214.

Adebamowo CA, et al. Milk consumption and acne in teenaged boys. *J Am Acad Dermatol.* 2008 May;58(5):787–793.

Al-Waili NS. Therapeutic and prophylactic effects of crude honey on chronic seborrheic dermatitis and dandruff. *Eur J Med Res.* 2001 Jul 30;6(7):306–308.

Bissett DL, Chatterjee R, Hannon DP. Photoprotective effect of superoxide-scavenging antioxidants against ultraviolet radiation-induced chronic skin damage in the hairless mouse. *Photodermatology, Photoimmunology and Photomedicine* 1990;7(2):56–62.

Boyce S, Supp A, Swope V, Warden G. Vitamin C regulates keratinocyte viability, epidermal barrier, and basement membrane in vitro and reduces wound contraction after grafting of cultured skin substitutes. *Journal of Investigative Dermatology.* 2002;118(4):565.

Chalmers RD, Kirby B. Gluten and psoriasis. *Br J Dermatol.* 2000;142: 5–7.

Danby FW. Diet and acne. *Clin Dermatol.* 2008 Jan–Feb;26(1): 93–96.

Filipiak B, Zutavern A, Koletzko S, Von Berg A, Brockow I, Grubel

A, et al. Solid food introduction in relation to eczema: results from a four-year prospective birth cohort study. *J Pediatr.* 2007;151: 352–358.

Galvan IJ, et al. Antifungal and antioxidant activities of the phytomedicine pipsissewa, *Chimaphila umbellata. Phytochemistry.* 2008 Feb;69(3):738–746. Epub. 2007 Oct 22.

Hayashi H, et al. Calorie restriction minimizes activation of insulin signaling in response to glucose: potential involvement of the growth hormone–insulin-like growth factor 1 axis. *Exp Gerontol.* 2008 Sep;43(9):827–832.

Henz BM, Jablonska S, Van De Kerkof PC, et al. Double-blind, multi-center analysis of the efficacy of borage oil in patients with atopic eczema. *Br J Dermatol.* 1999;140:685–688.

Katzman M, Logan AC. Acne vulgaris: nutritional factors may be influencing psychological sequelae. *Med Hypotheses.* 2007;69(5): 1080–1084.

Kharaeva Z, et al. Clinical and biochemical effects of coenzyme Q(10), vitamin E, and selenium supplementation to psoriasis patients. *Nutrition.* 2009 Mar 25(3):295–302.

Martindale S, McNeill G, Devereux G, Campbell D, Russell G, Seaton A. Antioxidant intake in pregnancy in relation to wheeze and eczema in the first two years of life. *Am J Respir Crit Care Med.* 2005;171:121–128.

Mrowietz U, Elder JT, Barker J. The importance of disease associations and concomitant therapy for the long-term management of psoriasis patients. *Arch Dermatol Res* 2006;298:309–319.

Norrman G, et al. Significant improvement of eczema with skin care and food elimination in small children. *Acta Paediatrica.* 2005;94:1384–1388.

Poulin Y, Bissonette R, Juneau C, Cantin K, Drouin R, Poubelle PE. XP-828L in the treatment of mild to moderate psoriasis: a randomized, double-blind, placebo-controlled study. *Alternative Medicine Review*. 2007;12(4): 352–359.

Purba MB, et al. Skin wrinkling: Can food make a difference? *J Am Coll Nutr*. 2001 Feb;20(1):71–80.

Reichrath J. Vitamin D and the skin: an ancient friend, revisited. *Exp Dermatol*. 2007 Jul;16(7):618–625.

Roshchupkin DI, Pistsov MY, Potapenko AY. Inhibition of ultraviolet light–induced erythema by antioxidants. *Arch Dermatol Res*. 1979;266:91–94.

Rubin MG, Kim K, Logan AC. Acne vulgaris, mental health, and omega-3 fatty acids: a report of cases. *Lipids Health Dis*. 2008 Oct 13;7:36.

Satchell AC, Saurajen A, Bell C, Barnetson RS. Treatment of dandruff with 5% tea tree oil shampoo. *J Am Acad Dermatol*. 2002 Dec;47(6):852–855.

Smith D, Kim YI, Refsum H. Is folic acid good for everyone? *Am J Clin Nutr*. 2008;87:517–533.

Smith RN, et al. The effect of a high-protein, low glycemic-load diet versus a conventional, high glycemic-load diet on biochemical parameters associated with acne vulgaris: a randomized, investigator-masked, controlled trial. *J Am Acad Dermatol*. 2007 Aug;57(2): 247–256.

Traub M, Marshall K. Psoriasis—pathophysiology, conventional, and alternative approaches to treatment. *Altern Med Rev*. 2007; 12(4):319–330.

www.healthy-skin-guide.com/foods-causing-eczema.html—last accessed 10/29/08.

www.mayoclinic.com/health/dandruff/DS00456/DSECTION
=causes—last accessed 11/11/08.

www.medicinenet.com/eczema/article.htm#tocc—last accessed 10/29/08.

www.medicinenet.com/seborrhea/article.htm—last accessed 11/03/08.

www.niams.nih.gov/Health_Info/Acne/acne_ff.asp#c—last accessed 11/12/08.

www.niapublications.org/agepages/skin.asp—last accessed 11/10/08.

www.sciencedaily.com/releases/2007/11/071109201438.htm—last accessed 11/10/08.

www.skincarephysicians.com/acnenet/acne.html—last accessed 11/12/08.

www.thedoctorsdoctor.com/diseases/acne_vulgaris.htm—last accessed 11/12/08.

Zulfakar MH, Edwards M, Heard CM. Is there a role for topically delivered eicosapentaenoic acid in the treatment of psoriasis? *Eur J Dermatol.* 2007 Jul–Aug;17(4):284–291.

Part 2: Go with the Flow

Resources

American Heart Association—www.americanheart.org

American Thyroid Association—http://thyroid.org

Raynaud's Association—www.raynauds.org

Mayo Clinic—www.mayoclinic.com/health/night-leg-cramps

National Institutes of Health—www.pubmedcentral.nih.gov/articlerender.fcgi?artid=1497008

Bibliography

Achike FI, Kwan CY. Nitric oxide, human diseases and the herbal products that affect the nitric oxide signalling pathway. *Clin Exp Pharmacol Physiol.* 2003;30(9):605–615.

Anselm E, et al. Grape juice causes endothelium-dependent relaxation via a redox-sensitive Src- and Akt-dependent activation of eNOS. *Cardiovasc Res.* 2007 Jan 15;73(2):404–413.

Armah CK, et al. Fish oil fatty acids improve postprandial vascular reactivity in healthy men. *Clin Sci* (Lond). 2008;114(11):679–686.

Chin-Dusting, JPF, et al. Effects of in vivo and in vitro L-arginine supplementation on healthy human vessels. *J Cardiovasc Pharmacol.* 1996;28:158–166.

Flammer AJ, et al. Dark chocolate improves coronary vasomotion and reduces platelet reactivity. *Circulation.* 2007;116(21):2376–2382.

Ignarro LJ, et al. Pomegranate juice protects nitric oxide against oxidative destruction and enhances the biological actions of nitric oxide. *Nitric Oxide.* 2006 Sep;15(2):93–102.

Pierce GL, et al. Weight loss alone improves conduit and resistance artery endothelial function in young and older overweight/obese adults. *Hypertension.* 2008;52(1):72–79.

Pittler MH, Ernst E. Horse chestnut seed extract for chronic venous insufficiency. *Cochrane Database Syst Rev.* 2006 Jan 25;(1).

Roffe C, Sills S, Crome P, Jones P. Randomised, cross-over, placebo-controlled trial of magnesium citrate in the treatment of chronic persistent leg cramps. *Med Sci Monit.* 2002;8(5):CR326–330.

Schindler R, Thöni H, Classen HG. The role of magnesium in the generation and therapy of benign muscle cramps. Combined in-vivo/in-vitro studies on rat phrenic nerve–diaphragm preparations. *Arzneimittelforschung.* 1998;48(2):161–166.

Schwellnus MP, Nicol J, Laubscher R, Noakes TD. Serum electrolyte concentrations and hydration status are not associated with exercise-associated muscle cramping (EAMC) in distance runners. *Br J Sports Med.* 2004;38(4):488–492.

Shi J, Yu J, Pohorly JE, Kakuda Y. Polyphenolics in grape seeds—biochemistry and functionality. *J Med Food.* 2003;6(4):291–299.

Part 3: House of Pain

Resources

National Migraine Association—www.migraines.org

National Headache Foundation—www.headaches.org

Mayo Clinic—www.mayoclinic.com/health/fibromyalgia

National Fibromyalgia Association—www.fmaware.org

Lupus Foundation of America—www.lupus.org

American Chronic Pain Association—www.theacpa.org

American Academy of Pain Management—www.aapainmanage.org

American Academy of Pain Medicine—www.painmed.org

Bibliography

Altura BM, Altura BT. Tension headaches and muscle tension: is there a role for magnesium? *Med Hypotheses.* 2001;57(6):705–713.

Amara S. Oral glutamine for the prevention of chemotherapy-induced peripheral neuropathy. *Ann Pharmacother.* 2008 Oct; 42(10):1481–1485.

Bic Z, Blix GG, Hopp HP, Leslie FM, Schell MJ. The influence of a low-fat diet on incidence and severity of migraine headaches. *J Womens Health Gend Based Med.* 1999;8:623–630.

Bloomer RJ, et al. Effects of antioxidant therapy in women exposed to eccentric exercise. *Int J Sport Nutr Exerc Metab.* 2004;14(4): 377–388.

Bryer SC, Goldfarb AH. Effect of high-dose vitamin C supplementation on muscle soreness, damage, function, and oxidative stress to eccentric exercise. *Int J Sport Nutr Exerc Metab.* 2006;16(3): 270–280.

Buettner C, et al. Prevalence of musculoskeletal pain and statin use. *J Gen Intern Med.* 2008;23(8):1182–1186.

Chariot P, Bignani O. Skeletal muscle disorders associated with selenium deficiency in humans. *Muscle Nerve.* 2003;27(6):662–668.

Cockburn E, et al. Acute milk-based protein–CHO supplementation attenuates exercise-induced muscle damage. *Appl Physiol Nutr Metab.* 2008;33(4):775–783.

Connolly DA, et al. Efficacy of a tart cherry juice blend in preventing the symptoms of muscle damage. *Br J Sports Med.* 2006; 40(8):679–683; discussion, 683.

Cunningham SM. Migraine: helping clients choose treatment and identify triggers. *Br J Nursing.* 1999; 8:1515–1523.

Gliottoni RC, Motl RW. Effect of caffeine on leg-muscle pain during intense cycling exercise: possible role of anxiety sensitivity. *Int J Sport Nutr Exerc Metab.* 2008;18(2):103–115.

Glore S, Ricker A. Trigeminal neuralgia: case study of pain cessation with a low-caffeine diet. *J Am Diet Assoc.* 1991;91(9): 1120–1121.

Hanington E. Migraine. In Lessof MH, ed., *Clinical reactions to food.* Chichester, UK: John Wiley, 1983:155–180.

Hoffman T. An ancient remedy and modern miracle drug. *Hawaii Med J.* 2007;66(12):326–327.

Lee P, Chen R. Vitamin D as an analgesic for patients with type 2 diabetes and neuropathic pain. *Arch Intern Med.* 2008;168(7): 771–772.

Lipton RB, Newman LC, Cohen JS, Solomon S. Aspartame as a dietary trigger of headache. *Headache.* 1989;29:90–92.

McCabe BJ. Dietary tyramine and other pressor amines in MAOI regimens: a review. *J Am Diet Assoc.* 1986;86:1059–1064.

Miller PC, Bailey SP, Barnes ME, Derr SJ, Hall EE. The effects of protease supplementation on skeletal muscle function and DOMS following downhill running. *J Sports Sci.* 2004;22(4):365–372.

Millichap JG, Yee MM. The diet factor in pediatric and adolescent migraine. *Pediatr Neurol.* 2003;28(1):9–15.

Peatfield RC. Relationships between food-, wine-, and beer-precipitated migrainous headaches. *Headache.* 1995;35:355–357.

Shimomura Y, et al. Nutraceutical effects of branched-chain amino acids on skeletal muscle. *J Nutr.* 2006;136(2):529S–532S.

Sima AA, Calvani M, Mehra M, Amato A; Acetyl-L-Carnitine Study Group. Acetyl-L-carnitine improves pain, nerve regeneration, and vibratory perception in patients with chronic diabetic neuropathy: an analysis of two randomized placebo-controlled trials. *Diabetes Care.* 2005;28(1):89–94.

Smith DJ, Olive KE. Chinese red rice–induced myopathy. *South Med J.* 2003;96(12):1265–1267.

www.merckmedicus.com/pp/us/hcp/diseasemodules/migraine /pathophysiology_sub.jsp—last accessed 11/06/08.

Part 4: It's All About Performance

Resources

American Heart Association—www.americanheart.org/presenter .jhtml?identifier=4644

Alzheimer's Association—www.alz.org

National Institute on Aging—www.nia.nih.gov; Building 31, Room 5C27, 31 Center Drive, MSC 2292, Bethesda MD 20892

WebMD—www.webmd.com/alzheimers/guide/alzheimers -dementia; www.webmd.com/anxiety-panic/default.htm

American Institute of Stress—www.stress.org

National Institutes of Health—www.nimh.nih.gov/health/topics /generalized-anxiety-disorder-gad/index.shtml

American Insomnia Association—www.americaninsomniaassociation .org

American Academy of Sleep Medicine—www.sleepeducation.com

The Andropause Society—www.andropause.org.uk

Everything Andropause—www.everythingandropause.com

Mayo Clinic—www.mayoclinic.org/bph; www.mayoclinic.com/health /low-sex-drive-in-women/DS01043; www.mayoclinic.com/health /menopause

BPH Health Forum—http://forum.urologychannel.com/hc-forum/bphenlarged-prostate_f206

Kidney Health—http://kidney.niddk.nih.gov/kudiseases/pubs/prostateenlargement

National Association for Continence—www.nafc.org

Urology Channel—www.urologychannel.com/prostate/bph/treatment_alt.shtml

Angela Grassi, MS, RD, LDN—www.pcosnutrition.com

American Fertility Association—www.theafa.org

Fertility Plus—www.fertilityplus.org

FDA—www.fda.gov/fdac/features/196_love.html

About.com—www.womenshealth.about.com/od/sexualdysfunction/Sexual_Dysfunction.htm; http://marriage.about.com/cs/lowsexdrive/a/2malelowlibido.htm

The National Women's Health Information Center—www.4woman.gov

North American Menopause Society (NAMS)—www.menopause.org

Bibliography

Adams PB, Lawson S, Sanigorski A, Sinclair AJ. Arachidonic acid to eicosapentaenoic acid ratio in blood correlates positively with clinical symptoms of depression. *Lipids.* 1996;31(Suppl):S157–161.

Afaghi A, O'Connor H, Chow CM. Acute effects of the very low carbohydrate diet on sleep indices. *Nutr Neurosci.* 2008 Aug;11(4):146–154.

Ajay Nehra, MD, FACS. Oral and non-oral combination therapy for erectile dysfunction. *Rev Urol.* 2007 Summer;9(3): 99–105.

Aoi W, et al. Exercise and functional foods. *Nutr J.* 2006;5:15.

Bansal TC, Guay AT, Jacobson J, et al. Incidence of metabolic syndrome and insulin resistance in a population with organic erectile dysfunction. *J Sex Med.* 2005;2:96–103.

Bent S, et al. Saw palmetto for benign prostatic hyperplasia. *N Engl J Med.* 2006;354(6):557–566.

Bosetti S, et al. Food groups and risk of prostate cancer in Italy. *Int J Cancer.* 2004;110:424–428.

Bravi F, Bosetti C, Dal Maso L, Talamini R, Montella M, Negri E, Ramazzotti V, Franceschi S, La Vecchia C. Macronutrients, fatty acids, cholesterol, and risk of benign prostatic hyperplasia. *Urology.* 2006;67(6):1205–1211.

Chyou PH, Nomura AM, Stemmermann GN, et al. A prospective study of alcohol, diet, and other lifestyle factors in relation to obstructive uropathy. *Prostate.* 1993;22:253–264.

Crispo R, et al. Alcohol and the risk of prostate cancer and benign prostatic hyperplasia, *Urology.* 2004;64 717–722.

Czeizel AE, Metneki J, Dudas I. The effect of preconceptional multivitamin supplementation on fertility. *Int J Vitam Nutr Res.* 1996;66:55–58.

Delion S, Chalon S, Guilloteau D, Besnard JC, Durand G. Alpha-linoleic acid dietary deficiency alters age-related changes of dopaminergic and serotoninergic neurotransmission in the rat frontal cortex. *J Neurochem.* 1996 Apr;66(4):1582–1591.

Denmark W, Robertson CN, Walther PJ, et al. Pilot study to explore effects of low-fat and flaxseed-supplemented diet on proliferation of benign prostatic epithelium and prostate specific antigen. *Urology.* 2004;63:900–904.

Dording CM, et al. A double-blind, randomized, pilot dose-finding study of maca root (*L. meyenii*) for the management of SSRI-induced sexual dysfunction. *CNS Neurosci Ther.* 2008 fall;14(3): 182–191.

Dorjgochoo T, et al. Dietary and lifestyle predictors of age at natural menopause and reproductive span in the Shanghai Women's Health Study. *Menopause.* 2008 Sep–Oct;15(5):924–933.

Duffy R, Wiseman H, File SE. Improved cognitive function in postmenopausal women after 12 weeks of consumption of a soya extract containing isoflavones. *Pharmacol Biochem Behav.* 2003 Jun;75(3):721–729.

Eby GA, Eby KL. Rapid recovery from major depression using magnesium treatment. *Med Hypotheses.* 2006;67(2):362–370.

Eskelinen MH, et al. Midlife coffee and tea drinking and the risk of late-life dementia: a population-based CAIDE study. *J Alzheimers Dis.* 2009 Jan;16(1):85–91.

Esposito K, Giugliano F, Di Palo C, et al. Effect of lifestyle changes on erectile dysfunction in obese men: a randomized controlled trial. *JAMA.* 2004;291:2978–2984.

Esposito K, Marfella R, Ciotola M, et al. Effect of a Mediterranean-style diet on endothelial dysfunction and markers of vascular inflammation in the metabolic syndrome: a randomized trial. *JAMA.* 2004;292:1440–1446.

Evans MF, MD. Lose weight to lose erectile dysfunction. *Can Fam Physician.* 2005 Jan 10;51(1):47–49.

Farshchi H, Rane A, Love A, Kennedy RL. Diet and nutrition in polycystic ovary syndrome (PCOS): pointers for nutritional management. *J Obstet Gynaecol.* 2007;27:762–773.

Fragakis SG, Thomson C. *The Health Professional's Guide to Popular Dietary Supplements, 3rd ed.* Chicago: American Dietetic Association, 2007:451–457.

Francis ST, Head K, Morris PG, Macdonald IA. The effect of flavanol-rich cocoa on the fMRI response to a cognitive task in healthy young people. *J Cardiovasc Pharmacol.* 2006;47 (Suppl 2):S215–220.

Galeone C, et al. Onion and garlic intake and the odds of benign prostatic hyperplasia. *Urology.* 2007;70(4):672–676.

Gass R. Benign prostatic hyperplasia: the opposite effects of alcohol and coffee intake. *BJU Int.* 2002;90(7):649–654.

Geller J, Sionit L, Partido C, et al. Genistein inhibits the growth of human-patient benign prostatic hyperplasia and prostate cancer in histoculture. *Prostate.* 1998;34:75–79.

Gillis CN. Panax ginseng pharmacology: a nitric oxide link? *Biochem Pharmacol.* 1997;54:1–8.

Heber D. Prostate enlargement: the canary in the coal mine? *Am J Clin Nutr.* 2002;75:605–606.

Heller E, Quinn T, Bussell JL. *Fully Fertile.* Chicago: Findhorn Press, 2008.

Hibbeln JR. Fish consumption and major depression. *The Lancet.* 1998;351(9110):1213.

Ho L, et al. Isolation and characterization of grape-derived polyphenolic extracts with Abeta-lowering activity that could be developed for Alzheimer's disease. Presented at Neuroscience 2007. San Diego, CA. Nov 3–7, 2007.

Ito TY, Polan ML, Whipple B, Trant AS. The enhancement of female sexual function with ArginMax, a nutritional supplement, among women differing in menopausal status. *J Sex Marital Ther.* 2006 Oct–Dec;32(5):369–378.

Johnston CS, Corte C, Swan PD. Marginal vitamin C status is associated with reduced fat oxidation during submaximal exercise in young adults. *Nutr Metab* (Lond). 2006 Aug 31;3:35.

Jorde R, Sneve M, Figenschau Y, Svartberg J, Waterloo K. Effects of vitamin D supplementation on symptoms of depression in overweight and obese subjects: randomized double-blind trial. *J Intern Med.* 2008 Dec;264(6):599–609.

Kalmijn S, et al. Dietary intake of fatty acids and fish in relation to cognitive performance at middle age. *Neurology.* 2004 Jan 27; 62(2):275–280.

Kim HS, Bowen P, Chen L, et al. Effects of tomato sauce on apoptotic cell death in prostate benign hyperplasia and carcinoma. *Nutr Cancer.* 2003;47:40–47.

Krikorian R, Nash TA, Shidler MD, Shukitt-Hale B, Joseph JA. Concord grape juice supplementation improves memory function in older adults. Presented at 37th Annual American Aging Association Meeting. Boulder, CO. May 30–June 2, 2008.

Kristal AR, et al. Dietary patterns, supplement use, and the risk of symptomatic benign prostatic hyperplasia: results from the prostate cancer prevention trial. *Am J Epidemiol.* 2008;167(8): 925–934.

Kupelian V, Shabsigh R, Araujo AB, et al. Erectile dysfunction as a predictor of the metabolic syndrome in aging men: results from the Massachusetts Male Aging Study. *J Urol.* 2006;176:222–226.

Lavialle M, et al. An (n-3) polyunsaturated fatty acid–deficient diet disturbs daily locomotor activity, melatonin rhythm, and striatal dopamine in Syrian hamsters. *J Nutr.* 2008;138:1719–1724.

Leathwood PD, Chauffard F, Heck E, et al. Aqueous extract of valerian root *(Valeriana officinalis L)* improves sleep quality in man. *Pharmacol Biochem Behav.* 1982;17:65–71.

Lehrl S. Clinical efficacy of kava extract WS 1490 in sleep disturbances associated with anxiety disorders. Results of a multicenter, randomized, placebo-controlled, double-blind clinical trial. *J Affect Disord.* 2004;78:101–110.

Liao S, Hiipakka RA. Selective inhibition of steroid 5 alpha reductase isozymes by tea epicatechin-3-gallate and epigallocatechin-3-gallate. *Biochem Biophys Res Commun.* 1995;214:833–838.

Lim SS, Noakes M, Norman RJ. Dietary effects on fertility treatment and pregnancy outcomes. *Curr Opin Endocrinol Diabetes Obes.* 2007 Dec;14(6):465–469.

Linde K, Berner M, Egger M, et al. St. John's Wort for depression: meta-analysis of randomised controlled trials. *Br J Psychiatry.* 2005;186:99–107.

Lucas M, et al. Ethyl-eicosapentaenoic acid for the treatment of psychological distress and depressive symptoms in middle-aged women: a double-blind, placebo-controlled, randomized clinical trial. *Am J Clin Nutr.* 2009 Feb;89(2):641–651.

Maughan RJ, et al. Diet composition and the performance of high-intensity exercise. *J Sport Sci.* 1997;15(3):265–275.

Minet-Ringuet J, Le Ruyet PM, Toméa D, Even PC. A tryptophan-rich protein diet efficiently restores sleep after food deprivation in the rat. *Behav Brain Res.* 2004;152:335–340.

Mizuno K, et al. Antifatigue effects of coenzyme Q10 during physical fatigue. *Nutrition.* 2008;24:293–299.

Moran LJ, Brinkworth GD, Norman RJ. Dietary therapy in polycystic ovary syndrome. *Semin Reprod Med.* 2008 Jan;26(1):85–92.

Morihara N, et al. Garlic as an anti-fatigue agent. *Molecular Nutrition and Food Research*. 2007;51(11):1329–1334.

Ng TP, et al. Curry consumption and cognitive function in the elderly. *Am J Epidemiol*. 2006 Nov 1;164(9):898–906.

Ng TP, et al. Tea consumption and cognitive impairment and decline in older Chinese adults. *Am J Clin Nutr*. 2008 Jul;88(1): 224–231.

Nozaki S, et al. Mental and physical fatigue–related biochemical alterations. *Nutrition*. 2009 Jan;25(1):51–57.

Nurk E, et al. Intake of flavonoid-rich wine, tea, and chocolate by elderly men and women is associated with better cognitive test performance. *J Nutr*. 2009;139(1):120–127.

Papandreou MA, et al. Effect of a polyphenol-rich wild blueberry extract on cognitive performance of mice, brain antioxidant markers, and acetylcholinesterase activity. *Behav Brain Res*. 2009 Mar 17;198(2):352–358.

Paschka, AG, Butler R, Young CY. Induction of apoptosis in prostate cancer cell lines by green tea component epigallocatechin-3-gallate. *Cancer Lett*. 1998;130:1.

Payne ME, Anderson JJ, Steffens DC. Calcium and vitamin D intakes may be positively associated with brain lesions in depressed and non-depressed elders. *Nutr Res*. 2008 May;28(5):285–292.

Pinelli G, Tagliabue A. Nutrition and fertility. *Minerva Gastroenterol Dietol*. 2007 Dec;53(4):375–382.

Pittler MH, Ernst E. Efficacy of kava extract for treating anxiety: systematic review and meta-analysis. *J Clin Psychol Pharmacol*. 2000 Feb; 20(1):84–89.

Richardson LK, Egede LE, Mueller M, Echols CL, Gebregziabher M. Longitudinal effects of depression on glycemic control in veterans with type 2 diabetes. *Gen Hosp Psychiatry.* 2008 Nov–Dec;30(6):509–514.

Rohrmann S, Giovannucci E, Willett WC, Platz EA. Fruit and vegetable consumption, intake of micronutrients, and benign prostatic hyperplasia in US men. *Am J Clin Nutr.* 2007;85(2):523–529.

Ruder EH, Hartman TJ, Blumberg J, Goldman MB. Oxidative stress and antioxidants: exposure and impact on female fertility. *Hum Reprod Update.* 2008 Jul–Aug;14(4):345–357. Epub 2008 Jun 4.

Schruers K, van Diest R, Overbeek T, et al. Acute L-5-hydroxytryptophan administration inhibits carbon dioxide–induced panic in panic disorder patients. *Psychiatry Res.* 2002; 113:237–243.

Shukitt-Hale B, Carey A, Simon L, Mark DA, Joseph JA. Effects of Concord grape juice on cognitive and motor deficits in aging. *Nutrition.* 2006;22(3):295–302.

Tanaka M, et al. Effects of (—)-epigallocatechin gallate in liver of an animal model of combined (physical and mental) fatigue. *Nutrition.* 2008 Jun;24(6):599–603.

Tanaka M, et al. Relationships between dietary habits and the prevalence of fatigue in medical students. *Nutrition.* 2008 Oct; 24(10):985–989.

Wertz K, Siler U, Goralczyk R. Lycopene: modes of action to promote prostate health. *Arch Biochem Biophys.* 2004;430:127–134.

Whittle N, Lubec G, Singewald N. Zinc deficiency induces enhanced depression-like behaviour and altered limbic activation reversed by antidepressant treatment in mice. *Amino Acids.* 2009 Jan;36(1):147–158.

Wilt T, Ishani A, MacDonald R, Rutks I, Stark G. *Pygeum africanum* for benign prostatic hyperplasia. *Cochrane Database Syst Rev. 2002;* (1): CD001044. DOI: 10.1002/14651858.CD001044.

Wilt T, Ishani A, MacDonald R, Stark G, Mulrow CD, Lau J. Beta-sitosterols for benign prostatic hyperplasia. *Cochrane Database Syst Rev.* 1999;(4):CD001043. DOI: 10.1002/14651858.CD001043.

Wlodek D, Gonzales M. Decreased energy levels can cause and sustain obesity. *J Theor Biol.* 2003 Nov 7;225(1):33–44.

www.emedicinehealth.com/insomnia—last accessed 09/13/08.

www.holisticonline.com/remedies/sleep/sleep_ins_food-and-diet.htm—last accessed 09/13/08.

www.medicinenet.com/menopause/page5.htm#tocm—last accessed 02/09/09

www.medicinenet.com/script/main/art.asp?articlekey=40606—last accessed 02/03/09.

www.naturalnews.com/020611.html—last accessed 08/09/08.

www.roystonclinic.com/Pages/Andropause.htm—last accessed 02/01/09.

www.webmd.com/anxiety-panic/guide/generalized-anxiety-disorder—last accessed 09/10/08.

Young SN. Folate and depression–a neglected problem. *J Psychiatry Neurosci.* 2007; 32(2):80–82.

Ziegler G, Ploch M, Miettinen-Baumann A, Collet W. Efficacy and tolerability of valerian extract LI 156 compound with oxazepam in the treatment of non-organic insomnia—a randomized, double-blind, comparative clinical study. *Eur J Med Res.* 2002;7: 480–486.

Part 5: Check Your Plumbing

Resources

American Academy of Family Physicians—http://familydoctor.org/online/famdocen/home/common/digestive/basic/037.html; http://familydoctor.org/online/famdocen/home/tools/symptom/534.html

Mayo Clinic—www.mayoclinic.com/health/diarrhea/DS00292; http://www.mayoclinic.com/invoke.cfm?id=DS00025

American Gastroenterological Association—www.gastro.org

American College of Gastroenterology—www.acg.gi.org

International Foundation for Functional Gastrointestinal Disorders—www.aboutgerd.org; www.aboutibs.org.

American Dental Association—www.ada.org/public/topics/bad_breath.asp#overview

www.gasmedic.com

www.flat-d.com

www.under-tec.com.

National Digestive Diseases Information Clearinghouse—http://digestive.niddk.nih.gov.

Mayo Clinic—www.mayoclinic.com/health/irritable-bowel-syndrome

International Foundation for Functional GI Disorders—www.iffgd.org

National Kidney Foundation—www.kidney.org

American Urological Association—www.urologyhealth.org

Bibliography

Adolfsson O. Yogurt and gut function. *Am J of Clin Nutr.* 2004; 80:245–256.

Albrecht U, Goos KH, Schneider B. A randomised, double-blind, placebo-controlled trial of a herbal medicinal product containing *Tropaeoli majoris herba* (nasturtium) and *Armoraciae rusticanae radix* (horseradish) for the prophylactic treatment of patients with chronically recurrent lower urinary tract infections. *Curr Med Res Opin.* 2007 Oct;23(10):2415–2422.

Apicella LL, Sobota AE. Increased risk of urinary tract infection associated with the use of calcium supplements. *Urol Res.* 1990;18:213–217.

Avorn J, Monane M, Gurwitz JH, Glynn RJ, Choodnovskiy I, Lipsitz LA. Reduction of bacteriuria and pyuria after injestion of cranberry juice. *JAMA.* 1994;271:751–754.

Barbara G, et al. Probiotics and irritable bowel syndrome: rationale and clinical evidence for their use. *J Clin Gastroenterol.* 2008;42:5214–5217.

Beyer PL. Medical nutrition therapy for lower gastrointestinal tract disorders. In Escott-Stump S, Mahan LK, eds. *Krause's Food, Nutrition, & Diet Therapy.* 11th ed. Philadelphia: WB Saunders, 2004:705–735.

Brandt LJ, et al. Systematic review on the management of chronic constipation in North America. *Am J Gastroenterol.* 2005; 100(Suppl 1):S5–21.

Broussard EK, Surawicz CM. Probiotics and prebiotics in clinical practice. *Nutr Clin Care.* 2004;7(3):104–113.

Canani RB, LoVecchio A, Guarino A. Probiotics as prevention and treatment for diarrhea. *Curr Opin Gastroenterol.* 2009 Jan; 25(1):18–23.

Chen HL, et al. Mechanisms by which wheat bran and oat bran increase stool weight in humans. *Am J Clin Nutr.* 1998;68:711–719.

Cummings JH, MacFarlane GT. Gastrointestinal effects of prebiotics. *Br J Nutr.* 2002;87(Suppl 2):S145–151.

De Paula JA, Carmuega E, Weill R. Effect of the ingestion of a symbiotic yogurt on the bowel habits of women with functional constipation. *Acta Gastroenterol Latinoam.* 2008;38:16–25.

Descrochers N, Brauer PM. Legume promotion in counseling: an e-mail survey of dietitians. *Can J Diet Prac Res.* 2001;62:193–198.

Dukas L, Willet WC, Giovannucci EL. Association between physical activity, fiber intake, and other lifestyle variables and constipation in a study of women. *Am J Gastroenterol.* 2003;98:1790–1796.

Fernandez-Banares F. Nutritional care of the patient with constipation. *Best Pract Res Clin Gasteroenterol.* 2006;20:575–587.

Gibson GR. Dietary modulation of the human gut microflora using the prebiotics oligofructose and inulin. *Am Socity Nutr Sci.* 1999; 129:1438S–1441S.

Jepson RG, Craig JC. A systematic review of the evidence for cranberries and blueberries in UTI prevention. *Mol Nutr Food Res.* 2007 Jun;52(6):738–745.

Kaltenbach T, Crockett S, Gerson L. Are lifestyle measures effective in patients with gastroesophageal reflux disease? *Arch Intern Med.* 2006;166:965–971.

Konturek SJ, et al. Protective influence of melatonin against acute esophageal lesions involves prostaglandins, nitric oxide and sensory nerves. *J Physiol Pharmacol.* 2007 Jun;58(2):361–377.

Lodhia P, et al. Effect of green tea on volatile sulfur compounds in mouth air. *J Nutr Sci* Vitaminol (Tokyo). 2008 Feb;54(1):89–94.

Nutrition Care Manual. American Dietetic Association. 2008. http://www.nutritioncaremanual.com—last accessed 02/10/09.

Nutrition Therapy for Gastroesophageal Reflux Disease. Nutrition Care Manual. American Dietetic Association. 2008. www .nutritioncaremanual.org.

Park M, Bae J, Lee DS. Antibacterial activity of [10]-gingerol and [12]-gingerol isolated from ginger rhizome against periodontal bacteria. *Phytother Res.* 2008 Sep 23;22(11):1446–1449.

Shi J, Tong Y, Shen JG, Li HX. Effectiveness and safety of herbal medicines in the treatment of irritable bowel syndrome: a systematic review. *World J Gastroenterol.* 2008 Jan 21;14(3):454–462.

Spiro HM. Fat, foreboding, and flatulence. *Ann Intern Med.* 1999;130:320–322.

Strate LL, Lui YL, Syngal S, Aldoori W, Giovannucci EL. Nut, corn, and popcorn consumption and the incidence of diverticular disease. *JAMA.* 2008;300:907–914.

Suvarna R, Pirmohamed M, Henderson L. Possible interaction between warfarin and cranberry juice. *BMJ.* 2003;327:1454.

Weiss EI, et al. Inhibiting interspecies coaggregation of plaque bacteria with a cranberry juice constituent *J Am Dent Assoc.* 1998 Dec;129(12):1719–1723.

www.webmd.com/food-recipes/news/20050310/yogurt-antidote-to-bad-breath—last accessed 11/01/08.

Yang G, Wu XT, Zhou Y, Wang YL. Application of dietary fiber in clinical enteral nutrition: a meta-analysis of randomized controlled trials. *World J Gastroenterol.* 2005;11(25):3935–3938.

Zuckerman, MJ. The role of fiber in the treatment of irritable bowel syndrome: therapeutic recommendations. *J Clin Gastroenterol.* 2006;40:104–108.

Part 6: A Good Foundation

Resources

National Osteoporosis Foundation—www.nof.org

National Institutes of Health—www.nlm.nih.gov/medlineplus /osteoporosis.html; http://nihseniorhealth.gov/osteoporosis/toc.html

The Arthritis Foundation—www.arthritis.org

American College of Rheumatology—www.rheumatology.org

National Institute of Arthritis and Musculoskeletal and Skin Diseases—www.niams.nih.gov

Mayo Clinic—www.mayoclinic.com/health/osteoarthritis

Bibliography

Ameye LG., Winnie SC. Osteoarthritis and nutrition. From nutraceuticals to functional foods: a systematic review of the scientific evidence. *Arthritis Res Ther.* 2006;8:R127.

Arjmandi BH, et al. Dried plums improve indices of bone formation in postmenopausal women. *J Womens Health Gend Based Med.* 2002 Jan–Feb;11(1):61–68.

Asinghe VJ, Perera CO, Barlow PJ. Bioavailability of vitamin D_2 from irradiated mushrooms: an in vivo study. *Br J Nutr.* 2005 Jun;93(6):951–955.

Battie MC, et al. 1991 Volvo Award in Clinical Sciences. Smoking and lumbar disc degeneration: an MRI study of identical twins. *Spine.* 1991;16:1015–1021.

Berbert AA, Kondo CR, Almendra CL, Matsuo T, Dichi I. Supplementation of fish oil and olive oil in patients with rheumatoid arthritis. *Nutrition.* 2005;21(2):131–136.

Boss GR, Ragsdale RA, Zettner A, Seegmiller JE. Failure of folic acid (pteroylglutamic acid) to affect hyperuricemia. *J Lab Clin Med.* 1980;96:783–789.

Butz DE, Li G, Huebner SM, Cook ME. A mechanistic approach to understanding conjugated linoleic acid's role in inflammation using murine models of rheumatoid arthritis. *Am J Physiol Regul Integr Comp Physiol.* 2007;293(2):R669–676.

Cashman KD. Altered bone metabolism in inflammatory disease: role for nutrition. *Proc Nutr Soc.* 2008; 67(2):196–205.

Choi HK, Atkinson K, Karlson EW, Curhan G. Obesity, weight change, hypertension, diuretic use, and risk of gout in men: The Health Professionals Follow-Up Study. *Arch Intern Med.* 2005; 165:742–748.

Choi HK, Atkinson K, Karlson EW, et al. Alcohol intake and risk of incident gout in men: a prospective study. *Lancet.* 2004;363: 1277–1281.

Choi HK, Atkinson K, Karlson EW, Willett W, Curhan G. Purine-rich foods, dairy and protein intake, and the risk of gout in men. *N Engl J Med.* 2004;350:1093–1103.

Choi HK, Curhan G. Beer, liquor, and wine consumption and serum uric acid level: The Third National Health and Nutrition Examination Survey. *Arthritis Care Res.* 2004; 51:1023–1029.

Choi HK, Curhan G. Soft drinks, fructose consumption, and the risk of gout in men: a prospective cohort study. *BMJ.* 2008; 336(7639):309–312.

Choi HK, Willett W, Curhan G. Coffee consumption and risk of incident gout in men: a prospective study. *Arthritis Rheum.* 2007; 56(6):2049–2055.

Cutolo M, Otsa K, Uprus M, Paolino S, Seriolo B. Vitamin D in rheumatoid arthritis. *Autoimmun Rev.* 2007;7(1):59–64.

Divine, A et al. Tea drinking is associated with benefits on bone density in older women. *Am J Clin Nutr.* 2007 Oct;86(4): 1243–1247.

Eaton-Evans J, et al. Dietary factors and vertebral bone density in perimenopausal women. *Proc Nutr Soc.* 1993;52:44A.

Edmonds SE, Winyard PG, Guo R, et al. Putative analgesic activity of repeated oral doses of vitamin E in the treatment of rheumatoid arthritis: results of a propective placebo-controlled, double-blind trial. *Ann Rheum Dis.* 1997;56(11):649–655.

Gaspardy G, Balint G, Mitsuova M, et al. Treatment of sciatica due to intervertebral disc herniation with Chymoral tablets. *Rheum Phys Med.* 1971;11:14–19.

Hak AE, Choi HK. Lifestyle and gout. *Curr Opin Rheumatol.* 2008;20(2):179–186.

Han A, Judd MG, Robinson VA, Taixiang W, Tugwell P, Wells G. Tai chi for treating rheumatoid arthritis. *Cochrane Database Syst Rev.* 2004;(3):CD004849. DOI: 10.1002/14651858.CD004849.

Hodgson J, et al. Chocolate consumption and bone density in older women. *Am J Clin Nutr.* 2008;87:175–180.

Jenkins DJ, Kendall CW, Vidgen E, Augustin LS, van Erk M, Geelen A, et al. High-protein diets in hyperlipidemia: effect of wheat gluten on serum lipids, uric acid, and renal function. *Am J Clin Nutr.* 2001;74:57–63.

Kiyohara C, Kono S, Honjo S, et al. Inverse association between coffee drinking and serum uric acid concentrations in middle-aged Japanese males. *Br J Nutr.* 1999; 82:125–130.

Kjeldsen-Kragh J. Rheumatoid arthritis treated with vegetarian diets. *Am J Clin Nutr.* 1999;70(Suppl 3):S594–600.

Lanham-New SA. The balance of bone health: tipping the scales in favor of potassium-rich, bicarbonate-rich foods. *Am J Clin Nutr J Nutr.* 2008;138:172S–177S.

Lanham-New SA. Importance of calcium, vitamin D, and vitamin K for osteoporosis prevention and treatment. *Proc Nutr Soc.* 2008;67(2):163–176.

Lin PH, et al. The DASH diet and sodium reduction improve markers of bone turnover and calcium metabolism in adults. *J Nutr.* 2003;133:3130–3136.

Macdonald HM, et al. Nutritional associations with bone loss during the menopausal transition: for a beneficial effect of calcium, alcohol, and fruit and vegetable nutrients and of a detrimental effect of fatty acids. *Am J Clin Nutr.* 2004;79:155–165.

MacLaughlin J, Holick MF. Aging decreases the capacity of human skin to produce vitamin D_3. *J Clin Invest.* 1985;76:1536–1538.

McAlindon TE, Felson DT, Zhang Y, Hannan MT, Aliabadi P, Weissman B, Rush D, Wilson PW, Jacques P. Relation of dietary intake and serum levels of vitamin D to progression of osteoarthritis of the knee among participants in the Framingham Study. *Ann Intern Med.* 1996;125(5):353–359.

McGartland CP, et al. Fruit and vegetable consumption and bone mineral density: the Northern Ireland Young Hearts Project. *Am J Clin Nutr.* 2004;80:1019–1023.

Michaelsson K, et al. Diet, bone mass, and osteocalcin: a cross-sectional study. *Calcif Tissue Int.* 1995;57:86–93.

Muhlbauer RC, Lozano A, Palacio S, Reinli A, Felix R. Common herbs, essential oils, and monoterpenes potently modulate bone metabolism. *Bone.* 2003;32:372–380.

Muhlbauer RC, Lozano A, Reinli A. Onion and a mixture of vegetables, salads, and herbs affect bone resorption in the rat by a mechanism independent of their base excess. *J Bone Miner Res.* 2002;17:1230–1236.

Pyrnne CJ, et al. Fruit and vegetable consumption and bone mineral status: a cross-sectional study across five age/gender cohorts. *Am J Clin Nutr.* 2006;83:1420–1428.

Roux C, et al. New insights into the role of vitamin D and calcium in osteoporosis management: an expert roundtable discussion. *Curr Med Res Opin.* 2008 May;24(5):1363–1370.

Tucker KL, et al. Colas, but not other carbonated beverages, are associated with low bone mineral density in older women: The Framingham Osteoporosis Study. *Am J Clin Nutr.* 2006 Oct;84(4): 936–942.

Vilim S, Vladimir K, Jitka U, Jiri GT. The efficacy of glucosamine and chondroitin sulfate in the treatment of osteoarthritis: are these saccharides, drugs, or nutraceuticals? *Biomed Papers.* 2005; 1:51–56.

Wim JB, et al. Glucosamine and chondroitin sulfate supplementation to treat symptomatic disc degeneration: biochemical rationale and case report. *BMC Complem Altern M.* 2003;3:2.

www.cinn.org/spine/disc-degeneration.html#causes—last accessed 09/28/08.

www.mayfieldclinic.com/pe-ddd.htm—last accessed 12/03/08.

www.med.umich.edu/1libr/guides/osteo.htm—last accessed 09/28/08.

www.webmd.com/back-pain/tc/degenerative-disc-disease-topic -overview—last accessed 09/28/08.

Part 7: Eyes on the Future

Resources

National Eye Institute (NEI)—www.nei.nih.gov

The American Academy of Ophthalmology—www.aao.org

The American Optometric Association—www.aoa.org

Macular Degeneration Foundation—www.eyesight.org

Foundation Fighting Blindness—www.blindness.org

The Lighthouse National Center for Vision and Aging—www .lighthouse.org

Prevent Blindness America—www.preventblindness.org

AMD Alliance International—www.amdalliance.org

Bibliography

Christen WG, et al. Folic acid, pyridoxine, and cyanocobalamin combination treatment and age-related macular degeneration in women: The Women's Antioxidant and Folic Acid Cardiovascular Study. *Arch Intern Med.* 2009 Feb 23;169(4):335–341.

Gale CR, et al. Plasma antioxidant vitamins and carotenoids and age-related cataract. *Ophthalmology.* 2001;108:1992–1998.

Jacques PF, et al. Long-term vitamin C supplement use and prevalence of early age-related lens opacities. *Am J Clin Nutr.* 1997; 66:911–916.

Krinsky NI, Landrum JT, Bone RA. Biologic mechanisms of the protective role of lutein and zeaxanthin in the eye. *Annu Rev Nutr.* 2003;23:171–201.

Mares-Perlman JA, et al. Vitamin supplement use and incident cataracts in a population-based study. *Arch Ophthalmol.* 2000; 118:1556–1563.

Moeller, et al. The potential role of dietary xanthophylls in cataract and age-related macular degeneration. *JACN.* 2000 Oct 19: 522S–527S.

Rhone M, Basu A. Phytochemicals and age-related eye diseases. *Nutr Rev.* 2008 Aug;66(8):465–472.

Seddon JM. Multivitamin-multimineral supplements and eye disease: age-related macular degeneration and cataract. *Am J Clin Nutr.* 2007 Jan;85(1):304S–307S.

Teikari JM, et al. Six-year supplementation with alpha-tocopherol and beta-carotene and age-related maculopathy. *Acta Ophthalmol Scand.* 1998;76:224–229.

West S, et al. Are antioxidants or supplements protective for age-related macular degeneration? *Arch Ophthalmol.* 1994;112: 222–227.

www.naturaldatabase.com—last accessed 09/22/08.

www.sciencedaily.com/releases/2008/08/080808104925.htm—last accessed 09/01/08.

INDEX

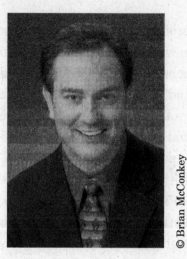

DAVID GROTTO, RD, LDN, is the president and founder of Nutrition Housecall, LLC, a nutrition consulting firm that provides nutrition communications, lecturing, and consulting services, and also offers personalized at-home dietary services.

David worked in the natural foods industry for more than twenty-five years; he owned and operated his own natural food store for more than eighteen of those years, which led him to become a registered dietitian. He graduated with honors from the University of Illinois at Chicago with a degree in medical dietetics and nutrition and was also bestowed the Excellence in Practice Award by the American Dietetic Association for his clinical work. He also served as a national spokesperson for the American Dietetic Association for more than six years.

For more than ten years he hosted his own live radio show, *Let's Talk Health, Chicago,* and also co-hosted the national television program *Health and Lifestyles Weekly.*

David serves on the scientific advisory board at *Fitness* magazine.

His acclaimed book *101 Foods That Could Save Your Life* (Bantam) has become the must-have food guide and reference for consumers and professionals alike. Dave also launched a video-centric companion website, www.101FoodsThatCouldSaveYourLife.com, which offers beautifully produced high-definition videos, additional recipes and tips, links to commodity and brand resources on the Web, and an online community where food and nutrition lovers can meet and interact.

One of Dave's passions is improving the health of children through good nutrition. He is the advisory board chair for Produce for Kids and the PBS Kids health initiative. Dave also lectures extensively on the benefits of humor and laughter therapy and is a Certified Laughter Leader; he has received further training in improvisation from the Second City in Chicago. He lives in the Chicagoland area with his wife, three daughters, and two dogs, which makes him an expert on the subject of "unopposed" estrogen.